Rukhmabai

Sudhir Chandra was formerly Senior Fellow, Centre for Social Studies, Surat, Gujarat and Visiting Professor, Institute for the Study of Languages & Cultures of Asia and Africa, Tokyo University of Foreign Studies. He is the author of *Gandhi: An Impossible Possibility* (2017), *Enslaved Daughters: Colonialism, Law and Women's Rights* (2008), *Continuing Dilemmas: Understanding Social Consciousness* (2002), *The Oppressive Present: Literature and Social Consciousness in Colonial India* (1992) and *Dependence and Disillusionment: Emergence of National Consciousness in Later 19th Century India* (1975).

Rukhmabai

The Life and Times of a
Child Bride Turned Rebel-Doctor

SUDHIR CHANDRA

MACMILLAN

First published in India 2024 by Macmillan
an imprint of Pan Macmillan Publishing India Private Limited
707 Kailash Building
26 K. G. Marg, New Delhi 110001
www.panmacmillan.co.in

Pan Macmillan, The Smithson, 6 Briset Street, Farringdon, London EC1M 5NR
Associated companies throughout the world
www.panmacmillan.com

ISBN 978-93-95624-61-9

Typeset in Arno Pro by R. Ajith Kumar, New Delhi
Printed in India by Gopsons Papers Pvt. Ltd., Noida

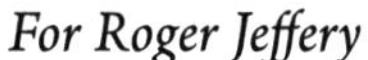

For Roger Jeffery

Contents

Preface

THIS BOOK PROVIDES GLIMPSES INTO the life and times of an extraordinary woman. As a young girl she came up, in absurdly unpropitious circumstances, with a radical notion of woman's freedom and fought for that notion. So radical was it that even our vaunted age of individual freedom and dignity has not realized it wholly. Her name – Rukhmabai – is a reminder of that unfinished momentous struggle.

She died a nonagenarian in 1955. But there is only a short phase of her long life for which a satisfactory body of information is available. This phase consists of the roughly twenty-five years between her mother's second marriage and her return as a doctor from the UK. Even that information, though, comes from secondary sources, such as court proceedings and newspapers reports. For the rest, barring random scraps of information, her biographer is crippled by near absence of primary material, and forced to tease out information from circumstantial evidence. There is complete absence of intimate personal documents like private letters, diaries, and memoirs which constitute the lifeblood of any biography.

One is required to make an enormous effort of imagination and also remember that, compared to fiction, biography permits imagination so much less leeway. To compensate for its scantiness, I have read the available material with the grain, against the grain, and between the lines. I have also ventured a leap, maybe two, with little more than speculation to show for evidence. The man who first showed me the way to do it is sociologist Paramjit Singh Judge. He showed it when I was writing on Rukhmabai's case. But I did not then have the courage to go all out.

Her name has in recent years come to be spelt as Rakhmabai. It has also been embellished with three surnames, none of which was ever used by her. For reasons that mattered to her, she presented herself all along as 'Rukhmabai'. That is how she was known during her lifetime and even posthumously. But in recent years, for reasons that matter to them, her biological descendants from her father and stepfather have sought to project her, respectively, as Save and Raut. Perhaps they do not know that neither her father, Janardan Pandurang, nor the stepfather, Sakharam Arjun, used any surname. The third surname given to her of late is Bhikaji. This is the most gratuitous of the three surnames. It shows, readers will soon see, that even as Rukhmabai is now an iconic figure, her iconicity is still lost on many. In any case, there can be no justification for meddling with the name she used for herself.

I have incurred numerous debts, big and small, in the course of writing this book. My biggest debt is to Roger Jeffery to whom the book is dedicated. With a generosity that is rare among scholars, he provided me endless information about Rukhmabai, especially for her years in London.

Antoinette Burton, Geraldine Forbes and Stephen Vitale, all of them familiar with Rukhmabai and her times, have helped me in a variety of ways. Muzaffar Alam sent me the scan of Mohini Varde's *Dr Rakhmabai: An Odyssey*. Manisha Chaudhary got me copies of research articles and books that I, with my Net illiteracy, could not have found on my own. Jose Burucua sent me the text of Nora Scott's *Journal*. Ambika Kulshreshtha was kind enough to translate Marathi passages for me. Leena Abraham sent me material from the Tata Institute of Social Science library. Shashank Sinha arranged to send some books. Abhinav Chandrachud provided some very useful information about judiciary in nineteenth-century India. Drs Ajoy Sodani and Aparna Sodani helped me understand the niceties of Rukhmabai's medical training and expertise. Dr Ketan Shelat and Dr Dharmesh Mehta, both associated with the Sheth Morarbhai Vijbhukhandas Hospital – now popularly known as the Rukhmabai Hospital – showed me around the building where Rukhmabai lived and worked for twenty-odd years, and also showed me some interesting photographs, besides giving a copy of a commemorative brochure about the Hospital.

Mridula Ramanna, whose work on Western medicine and healthcare in colonial Bombay is seminal, has been very supportive. She also put me in touch with her student, Dr Shubha Pandya, who passed on a good deal of information about Dr Atmaram Pandurang. So did Shri Deepak Mehta.

Makrand Mehta provided information about the first hospital for women in Ahmedabad.

Tridip Suhrud, like only he can, helped me acquire necessary information about Rukhmabai's days in Rajkot.

Gyan Pandey went through and edited portions of the book, and provided valuable suggestions.

I must also acknowledge the help received from Arvind Ganachari, Raja Dixit and Ashok Pawar.

To all these people – and to those I am failing to recall now – my deepest gratitude.

The entire book has been written under Jayanti Pandey's hospitable roof. I feel overwhelmed by her love, care, generosity and concern.

And, finally, my gratitude to Teesta Guha Sarkar. She felt it as a call of duty to offer the world a biography of Rukhmabai and made me her instrument.

S. C.

Introduction

MORE OFTEN THAN WE SUSPECT, entry of individuals and events into history depends on chance. In 1967, just twelve years after Rukhmabai's death, I was advised to consult the personal library of Dr Sakharam Arjun for my doctoral dissertation on the emergence of national consciousness in India. The descendants of Dr Sakharam – the gracious Rauts – welcomed me to their distinguished ancestor's library. I worked in their late nineteenth-century colonial-style bungalow – now a heritage site – for nearly a fortnight. However, neither those who had advised me to work there nor those living in the bungalow so much as mentioned Rukhmabai or told me that the bungalow had been built by her mother. Rukhmabai had not yet entered history.

What, eventually in 1975, led me to her was a chance discovery. I was working at the Nehru Memorial Museum & Library for a paper on the founding of the Indian National Social Conference in 1887. I had decided to begin by reading the issues of the *Indian Spectator* from the January of 1887 onwards to see when the idea of the Conference was first publicly mooted. I had just entered the first week of March when I ran into an editorial on the Rukhmabai case.

I read the editorial in wondrous disbelief. Here was a young woman in her early twenties refusing to cohabit with a husband she said she disliked. Daring the unthinkable, she had challenged, simultaneously, the mightiest two in the land – the British Indian legal system and entrenched Hindu orthodoxy. Instantly, the Indian National Social Conference was forgotten. As disbelief transformed into awed joy, I ransacked all the relevant newspapers and journals available at the Nehru Library. That done, I turned to the material available at the National Archives.

This preliminary research led to my first paper on Rukhmabai and her case. Presented in 1976 at a seminar on dissent, protest and reform in Indian civilization at the Indian Institute of Advanced Study, the paper appeared the following year in a volume comprising the proceedings of the seminar.[1]

This was, arguably, Rukhmabai's maiden independent entry into contemporary academic discourse. She had earlier found occasional passing mentions in biographies of some of the eminent public figures of the day who had, depending on their sociocultural orientations, supported or opposed her cause. These mentions were meant by the respective biographers to valorize their protagonists. No matter whether the mention meant praising or criticizing Rukhmabai, little interest was shown in understanding even the basic facts of her case. For instance, referring to Rukhmabai's marriage with Dadaji Bhikaji, and describing her as Dr Sakharam Arjun's daughter, Richard P. Tucker writes in his otherwise reliable *Ranade and the Roots of Indian Nationalism*:

> The father refused to send Rukhmabai to Dadaji during his own lifetime, since she was still a young girl. When he died, leaving her a considerable inheritance, Dadaji asked the courts to compel her to live with him … A lower court upheld Rukhmabai on the grounds that she had married Dadaji without her consent and hitherto could not be forced to live with him … The Rukhmabai controversy ended late in 1887 when Dadaji decided not to pursue his claims against his wife …[2]

Relying primarily on James Kellock's biography of Ranade, Tucker's account is not only replete with errors, it also minimizes Rukhmabai's travails and, consequently, her courage, bravery and determination. To that we shall turn later.

To return to the 1976 seminar at the Indian Institute of Advanced Study, no one there had ever heard of Rukhmabai. Indeed, even as late as 1984, Rukhmabai was virtually unknown not only among historians of colonial India but also among the fast-emerging feminists. I was speaking on the Rukhmabai case at a conference organized by Veena Mazumdar under the auspices of her newly founded Women's Studies Centre. Here, too, no one – not even the feminist participants – knew of Rukhmabai or her case. In the early 1990s I devoted myself exclusively to extensive research on the Rukhmabai case. A paper of mine, 'Whose Laws? Notes on a Legitimising Myth of the Colonial Indian State', appeared in 1992, and another, 'Rukhmabai: Debate over Woman's Right over Her Person', in 1996.[3] Finally, in 1998, I published an entire book on the subject, *Enslaved Daughters: Colonialism, Law and Women's Rights*.

Rukhmabai now is an iconic figure.

She was not when I spoke about her at the Women's Studies Centre's maiden seminar. In fact, it was with astonished elation that the feminists gathered there heard about this unknown forebear of theirs. As they listened to Rukhmabai's extraordinary defiance and Justice Pinhey's extraordinary verdict in her favour, they were struck by the uncanny resemblance between her case and, a whole century later, the Saritha case (1983) which had ended with Justice Chaudhury's stirring judgment in her favour.

If the feminists were innocent of the epochal drama of the 1880s, I was unaware of its repetition in my own day. For me, at least, the interaction with feminists proved most beneficial, as is evident from *Enslaved Daughters*. But for this interaction, I could not have grasped that what I believed was a moment in the history of colonial India has still not spent itself. It continues to dog us into the eighth decade of our independence. The dream Rukhmabai dreamt of women's dignity and rights remains unrealized in matters that are of vital concern to humans.

The appreciation of what she envisioned has been strangely tardy and partial. Even when she began to attract academic – especially feminist academic – attention during the 1990s, the heart of her defiance was missed. She was misrepresented as one seeking divorce. The opening paper in the inaugural number of the *Indian Journal of Gender Studies* (1994) describes Rukhmabai as one 'who was well known for her court case for divorce (the first ever in India)'.[4] Four years later, the otherwise well-researched *At the Heart of the Empire: Indians and the Colonial Encounter in Late-Victorian Britain* wrote of 'Rukhmabai, whose Bombay divorce case filled the metropolitan and provincial newspapers in Britian between 1884 and 1888'.[5] In fact, the first to so misrepresent the Rukhmabai case was the no less meticulous Tanika Sarkar, who wrote in 1993: 'Rukma Bai belonged to the carpenter's caste where divorce had been customary. Whose laws must colonial law recognise now?' Also: 'A lot of debate centred around the vexed question – whether a women [sic] could sue for separation from an adulterous husband.'[6]

In a doubly surprising persistence of the belief that Rukhmabai's was a case of divorce, Swati Save writes: 'I am sharing her [Rukhmabai's] odyssey ... because of her grueling experience and journey during her divorce back in 1880 when women in Indian tradition were going on pyre with their dead husbands, a system called as "sati" ... Divorcing someone you didn't approve was not dared in those days. Rukhamabi's divorce was the first divorce in India in 1880.'[7] Leaving aside the women going on pyre with their dead husbands, the persistence of the divorce myth in Save is doubly surprising because it appeared in 2012, by when so much was known about Rukhmabai; and because it came from one who, as a descendant of Janardan Pandurang, Rukhmabai's biological father, should have known at least the essentials of her illustrious ancestor's case.

Rukhmabai's was a suit for the restitution of conjugal rights. Divorce had nothing to do with it. The court at no point was called upon to consider whether divorce was customarily permitted among the carpenters, the community to which the litigants belonged. Nor was adultery relevant to the case. Adultery did come up in the course of the litigation, but it related to Narayan Dhurmaji, the maternal uncle of Dadaji under whose roof he was living. Also, Rukhmabai did say in a private letter, made public by the London *Times*, that Dadaji had gone 'through every course of dissipation' in 'ways which a woman's lips cannot utter'.[8] Adultery may well have been part of that unutterable litany of dissipation. But it did not figure in Rukhmabi's defence against Dadaji's restitution claim.

A case of divorce needs must recognize the marriage from which it seeks release. Rukhmabai was way more radical. She was denying the very marriage that had occasioned the suit against her. And she was doing so on high principles. Her initial defence did cite specific circumstances, such as incompatibility, the rotten state of her husband's health, and his inability to maintain her. But soon her defence came to rest entirely on principles, not on specific merits.

The principles Rukhmabai proclaimed still await full judicial and legislative acceptance. And that wait has exceeded a hundred and thirty years.

If the misconception that hers was a case of divorce downplays the principles she stood for, there is another misconception that downplays the enormity of her suffering. This comprises the belief that her marriage was dissolved by Victoria, the Queen-Empress. It figures particularly prominently in many internet accounts about Rukhmabai.[9] These accounts, sadly, inform public opinion more than does academic discourse these days. Indeed, they are getting into academic discourse as well. An attenuated variant of the belief regarding Victoria's benign intervention on behalf of Rukhmabai has, in fact, become part of academic discourse. Referring to Rukhmabai's awesome avowal that she would rather undergo the maximum penalty admissible under the law than obey the court's decree to go to her husband, Tanika Sarkar writes: 'The threat [of Rukhmabai's imprisonment] was removed only after considerable reformist agitation and the personal intervention of Victoria.'[10]

Contrast this with the actual effect of Rukhmabai's avowal. On 30 March 1887, even as the reformers were squabbling over how to save her, and before Victoria could be apprised of the happenings in the Bombay High Court, Viceroy Dufferin worriedly cabled his Law Member, Andrew Scoble: 'I hope you are keeping your eye on the Rukhmabai case. It will never do to allow her to be put into prison.'[11] The same day, not knowing how anxious on his own the Viceroy was, the Bombay government prayed to him for prompt remedial action.[12]

No less worried that Rukhmabai might really manage to get into prison and discredit the Hindu orthodoxy, Bal Gangadhar Tilak used his weeklies, the Marathi *Kesari* and the English *Mahratta*, to warn that the decree against Rukhmabai should not be enforced. Lest this be seen as a sign of defeat, it was asked if a woman like Rukhmabai was worth living with.

Dadaji Bhikaji was but a puny pawn in the momentous legal war that Rukhmabai was engaged in. Her real antagonists were the imperial government and the Hindu orthoxy. Exposed to serious loss of face by her defiance, both were looking for a way out.

The moral grandeur of Rukhmabai's act is diminished by the unfounded belief that Queen Victoria's intervention helped her avoid imprisonment. Equally diminishing and unfounded is the belief that her marriage was graciously annulled by Victoria. The pragmatic British reluctance to meddle with their Indian subjects' socio-religious affairs apart, the Queen-Empress had no authority to annul a Hindu marriage. In what is among the most sombre aspects of her case – as we shall see – Rukhmabai knew, and told the court, that, unlike the man suing her, she would not be entitled to marry again.

If there are misconceptions that diminish the grandeur of Rukhambai's defiance, there also are others that unduly magnify the enormity of her plight. She is represented, for example, as demanding 'to be released from a marriage contracted in infancy'.[13] Both in the late nineteenth century public discourse and in subsequent historiography a clear distinction figures between infant marriage and child marriage. Rukhmabai's plight was bad enough for being married at or around eleven. It was also reason enough to press for social and legislative reform. But she was not a victim of infant marriage.

Scholarship on Rukhmabai betrays, like she herself did all her life, another misconception which has serious civilizational implications. It is often believed that Hindu law – whatever the term is presumed to mean – enabled Rukhmabai's husband to drag her to a court of law to enforce his conjugal rights. This misconception has been best memorialized in the following damning ditty by Rudyard Kipling:

Graduate reformers with an English Education –

Lights of Aryavarta take our Heartiest applause,

For the spectacle you offer of an 'educated' nation.

Working out its freedom under 'educated' laws...

You can lecture government, draught a resolution...

Never such an opening for touching elocution

As the text of Rukhmibai, jailed by Hindu law.

What? No word of protest? Not a sign of pity?

Not a hand to help the girl, but, in black and white

Writes the leading oracle of the leading city:

'We the Indian nation, *we* hold it served her right.'[14]

It is easy to understand Swati Save's hagiographic portrayal of Rukhmabai. The proud descendant has happily taken in, with all its embellishments, the family's lore about their illustrious ancestor. Even Kipling's account can be explained. The herald of the White Man's Burden believed the 'Natives' were naturally degenerate. Except that, as an intelligent and sensitive young man who had closely covered the *Dadaji Bhikaji vs Rukhmabai* case, he should have remembered Justice Pinhey's indictment that the law relating to restitution of conjugal rights was a barbarous English importation into India; and that Hindu law contained no provision for imprisonment in matrimonial cases.

What really baffles is that serious scholarship should be vitiated by unfounded misconceptions. I have agonized over whether I should state the harsh truth. To do that is embarrassing because my own work is involved. However, since I have undertaken to write this biography, I must risk the embarrassment. Most of those who have considered Rukhmabai important enough for inclusion in their writing have written without doing serious research on her. It is no mere coincidence that misconceptions like her case having been one of divorce disappeared from scholarly writing following the publication of *Enslaved Daughters*. That is not a book about Rukhmabai. It is centred around her case. It has only one chapter, 'Rukhmabai and Her Case', that provides a basic biographical perspective. This chapter, courtesy some altruistic academic institution, has for long been available on the internet. Freed from the confines of the book, the accessibility of the chapter has increased manifold, and it appears to have become the source from which the more serious-minded derive information about Rukhmabai.

Things could have been different without the hegemonic presence of English in our academic discourse. In 1981, five years after my first paper on Rukhmabai, a grand-niece of hers, Mohini Varde, brought out *Dr Rakhmabai: Ek Aart*, a biography in Marathi. This was followed two years later by Sarojini Sharangpani's *Mala He Lagna Many Nahi*, a Marathi novel on Rukhmabai. But, as evidenced by Rukhmabai's case being described till the 1990s as one of divorce, even Marathi-knowing scholars used neither the biography nor the novel. The easiest access was, still is, to *Enslaved Daughters* and the chapter uploaded on the internet.

But now I can see – and this should erase the impression of egotism on my part – that even the little biographical information provided in *Enslaved Daughters* is not unflawed. For all the comprehensive research and close reading that went into the book, it is an unabashed celebration of an epochal resistance. A subtle bias, consequently, runs through the book. In that Rukhmabai was the one who dared that resistance, the bias may seem to stem from unabashed admiration for her. The admiration in the book is actually for the cause that Rukhmabai braved to embody. That admiration caused me to, unwittingly, judge Rukhmabai herself harshly at the slightest suspicion of failing the cause. A feeling verging on hostility possessed me when I learnt that she began to dress like a widow after the death of the man she had refused to recognize as her husband. It took me long – that's a separate story – to see Rukhmabai as a person, not an idealized embodiment of women's cause.

When this could happen to Rukhmabai in the event she got pitted against the Rukhmabai my imagination had conjured into existence, an even stronger bias against her adversaries and critics entered the book. In weighing their testimonies and narratives against those of Rukhmabai and her supporters, I forgot the first truth about court proceedings. I forgot, with regard to Rukhmabai and her defence, that litigation invariably induces an entire spectrum of inexactitudes that can range from carefully crafted ambiguities to plain lies.

The historian in me was not quite asleep in *Enslaved Daughters*. Yet, the subtly operating inclination to suspect those opposed to Rukhmabai resulted in a biographical sketch that now appears suspect. Closer re-examination of conflicting claims and narratives may alter even basic facts, like dates of birth and marriage, provided in the book. This is what, among other things, this biography attempts to do.

There is, however, a greater reason for the biography. I stated in *Enslaved Daughters*:

> The story possesses more hermeneutic possibilities than I have followed in this monograph, or am even aware of. Rukhmabai, to cite what may seem a striking lacuna, could have been a more pervasive and direct presence. Closer attention to biographical details could have revealed the psycho-social factors that gave her the strength to rebel where most women submitted to or chose less defiant ways of negotiating a similar suffering.[15]

The book, I had hoped, would act as a provocation for further exploration, especially by women scholars. My stress on a woman writing a book on Rukhmabai had emerged from a desired dialectic between the ideological and the existential. As a man writing on Rukhmabai, and living with her at the same time that I was living with my fiction writer spouse, I had begun aspiring to be, also, a woman; without forgetting the shadow that falls, always, between aspiring and being. It was akin to Deirdre David's desire in *Intellectual Women and Victorian Patriarchy*:

> I would like to think a male critic could have written this book, or perhaps, should say would have wanted to do so. For me, the desire of female and male critics to write from a feminist perspective about writers of both sexes signifies an end to the patriarchal attitudes resisted in one way or another, by Martineau, Browning and Eliot.[16]

Many women have since written on Rukhmabai without making her central to their work. The kind of explorations I had hoped for have not materialized. Meanwhile, I have myself been provoked by Pan Macmillan to attempt what I had provoked others to do. There is an urgent need for a biography of Rukhmabai in English. The only book in English that could pass for a biography is *Dr Rakhmabai: An Odyssey*. An indifferent translation of the Marathi biography by Rukhmabai's grand-niece, this book is, sadly, unavailable in the market and scarcely available in libraries. Though not uninformed like Save's panegyric, the *Odyssey* is in the category of proud descendants' narratives of their illustrious ancestors.

Biographers of the eminent of colonial India are forced to make do with agonizingly scant sources. One attempting a biography of Rukhmabai has nothing of the lively memoirs – her own or about her – telling anecdotes, diaries and private correspondence that constitute the staple of an engaging biography. There is plenty of varied material relating to her case which, read between the lines, can yield unexpected insights into her personal life. The same can be done through similarly reading the few letters to the press and articles that she wrote. For the rest, one has to cull out information from writings about related persons, movements, events and institutions. The only exception, perhaps, is Cornelia Sorabji, a contemporary of Rukhmabai, in whose case a rich atypical family archive enabled a gifted nephew to produce a comprehensive biography.[17]

Returning to entry into history being a game of chance, it is often asked: Why, despite having lived into our own day, did Rukhmabai have to wait an entire century to enter the annals? And a gendered answer is offered. Forgetting that it was a male who ushered her into the annals. Be that as it may, having spent more of my time in the second half of the nineteenth century than in the two subsequent centuries that I have physically inhabited, I can vouch that Rukhmabai is not an isolated victim – and beneficiary – of chance in history. There is an embarrassingly long list of forgotten greats – male and female – who are waiting for a propitious moment to enter history. Their wait may never end.

1

Beginnings in Sadness

SAD – *UDAS* IN MORE INDIAN languages than one – sums up Rukhmabai's life. There are two photographs of this pioneer fighter for women's rights. One, taken in a studio, is from her youth. Her right arm resting on a pedestal coming up to her waist, she stands elegantly in a gorgeous broad-bordered nine-yard silk sari and a loose full-sleeved blouse, a necklace peeping from under her *pallu*, a tiny dot adorning the centre of her forehead, and tops in her ears. The other photograph, taken at home, is from her old age. Wearing a plain sari and a full-sleeved blouse – both white, a colour that later in this narrative will tell a poignant tale – she is lean, tall, and elegant, presenting the very picture of graceful ageing. What defines her in both these photographs – all through her long life – is sadness.

There is yet another, little known, photograph of her youth which was taken in a London studio and published in the *Woman's Signal* of 25 October 1894. This one, like the other two, confirms what an English lady wrote after meeting Rukhmabai in March 1887: 'Her fine intelligent face had a tinge of sadness in it, and her manner, though cordial and pleasant, was very quiet.'[1]

Rukhmabai attributed the miseries of her life to her marriage. That happened when she was only eleven, and it would plague her all through the eighty or so years she lived thereafter. But even in the few years before that life-marring event, she knew no happiness. The first blow was struck when she was a toddler.

Let us begin from the beginning. Rukhmabai was the only child of Jayantibai and Janardan Pandurang. Janardan was a propertied man. He had inherited a house from his father, Tirthroop Pandurang Manikji, and to that he had added more property from his own earnings as a contractor. It comprised a 'dwelling house and a chawl', 'another house', and the moiety of a 'house and a garden.' The entire property was worth around twenty-five thousand rupees, a considerable fortune those days.

Rukhmabai was two-and-a-half when Janardan died, leaving her an orphan. Fortunately, however, Jayantibai's father, Harishchandra Yadavaji – Harichand Jadowji in contemporary accounts – brought his seventeen-year-old widowed daughter and little granddaughter to stay with him. Also, fortunately, just days before his death in 1867, Janardan had hastened to make a will, bequeathing his property to Jayantibai and assuring her of a regular income. He had also, in his will, nominated Harishchandra as the custodian of the property. This was to protect Jayantibai from the familiar phenomenon of widows being cheated by their deceased husband's unscrupulous relatives.

Harishchandra himself was a reasonably well-off man of good repute. A minor official in the Public Works Department, he had built for himself a fine house in the vicinity of the French Bridge, a respectable address in Bombay. He would later be appointed a Justice of the Peace and honoured by the government with the title of Rai Bahadur.

Harishchandra had the means and the will to make life happy for his hapless daughter and granddaughter. But he could get them little more than material security. He had remarried after the death of his first wife, from whom Jayantibai was born. To this second wife her step-daughter and step-granddaughter were unwelcome intruders: two unwanted mouths to feed, and as many competitors for her husband's attention. Making sure that not a word went unheard, she would every day curse her ill stars for inflicting on her happy family the inauspicious widow and her brat. Little Rukhmabai grew up watching her mother suffer. Worse, not knowing why, she would herself become the object of her step-grandmother's ire. Even more baffling and unbearable would be to have directed at her the harassed mother's pent-up frustration and anger. Yet, in tender irony, the helpless child would try and comfort, like only a child can, her helpless mother in the solitude of night.

Destined not to have a child of her own, Rukhmabai, as a young girl, had become mother to her suffering mother. Soon she would be mothering her remarried mother's children. To that searing irony we will come shortly.

In the little she wrote about her life, Rukhmabai maintained an impenetrable silence about her six dark years at Harishchandra's. Except for a passing poignant mention of the bereavement that left her an orphan. That done, she moved straightaway to her life under her stepfather's roof. There is little doubt, though, that her growing into a sad, introverted and precocious girl had its origins in the stress, shame and agony of those years. As had her sceptical view of family and society.

Things could have become messier had Jayantibai succumbed to her husband's dying wish. He had, characteristically for his times, willed that Jayantibai 'is to adopt, with the consent of my executor, a good son for the purpose of my ancestors' name'. She may have had her weaker moments. But Harishchandra, the will's executor, had willed to not let his daughter remain a widow all her life. Fortunately, widow marriage was a common practice in his community of Suthars. He began persuading Jayantibai to start a new life, and searching for a suitable man. The search lasted six years and the choice was worth the long wait.

It was the thirty-four-year-old Dr Sakharam Arjun, a distinguished doctor and botanist who had already made a mark in the public life of Bombay for, among other things, his advocacy of social reform. Born in a poor family and orphaned when he was eleven, Sakharam was a self-made man. He was not even thirty when his first wife died. For nearly five years he parried his mother's pestering to remarry, keeping at bay prospective fathers-in-law who were all keen to make the worthy widower their son-in-law.

It was assumed that the eminent doctor would remarry sooner rather than later. Also that, in keeping with the times and his mother's insistence, he would marry a nubile virgin. The prevailing practice was for respectable males to have a virgin wife. Old widowers and polygamists too wanted virgin wives. There was even a group of social reformers that approved of remarriage only for virgin widows, not for those whose marriage had been consummated. This selective advocacy of widow marriage sprang from a deep-seated horror of marrying a woman whom another male had 'known'.

That horror is writ large in the stark reference to the vagina of the prospective bride: *akshat* and *kshat yoni* – unpenetrated as opposed to penetrated vagina. Only a widow whose vagina had not been penetrated was supposed to be eligible for remarriage. The terms also point to a deep-seated patriarchal possessiveness, an obsession with monopolizing the sexuality of their woman/women.

Understandably, then, while the parleys for marriage with Sakharam were on, Jayantibai was consumed by the anxiety of whether the debonair doctor would consent to marry a widow with whom would come her eight-and-a-half-year-old daughter. Jayantibai was in for a happy shock. Sakharam proved exceptionally true to his commitment to social reform. For, precisely when he married a twenty-three-year-old widowed mother, the star social reformer of the day, Mahadev Govind Ranade, aged thirty-one, succumbed to his father's pressure and married a previously unmarried eleven-year-old girl. And married her within barely a month of his first wife's death.

There is an unlikely romantic detail about the Jayantibai–Sakharam union. Agonizing that she might be rejected, she did the inconceivable. Disregarding possible ridicule, she sent Sakharam a letter, saying she wished to be his life partner. The doctor, chivalrously, chose the daring lady.

From the look of it, eight-and-a-half-year-old Rukhmabai could not have got a better stepfather. Being under his roof and care was sure to bring her relief from the cheerless and fearful existence of the preceding six years. She and her mother would have a home – a grand one – of their own, rid forever of the searing glares and invectives of Yadavaji's second wife. Best, the stepfather was a thorough advocate of female education. At a time when elementary schooling was believed to be all that was required for girls, Sakharam was convinced:

> Do we really believe that the mere smattering of learning given to our girls in the vernacular schools is sufficient for the regeneration of India? These schools have been doing well in their own way, but shall we stop here in case of women, when not only we, also everything around us is rapidly advancing? ... is it not a fact that nine out of every ten unlearn, as wives and mothers, what they learnt as girls? But even if they retained in afterlife what they picked up at these primary schools, will that help them much to become efficient wives and mothers? I am afraid not. They want higher education, which would develop and inform their minds.[2]

Jayantibai and Rukhmabai were in a home of their own, with a man than whom they could not have got, respectively, a better husband and a better stepfather. For Rukhmabai, in fact, this would be her first experience of home after the shame and helplessness of six years of their dependence. Of course, here too, there was a peeved step-grandmother to contend with. But she, compared to the maternal step-grandmother left behind, was unlikely to be worse than a minor irritant. Disappointed to have got a daughter-in-law with whom had come her eight-and-a-half-year-old daughter, she was not going to easily warm up to them. But she could be expected to avoid needless friction within the family.

All told, life at Sakharam's seemed to promise well.

Then, out of the blue, everything changed. Sakharam married Rukhmabai off at eleven. Were it Jayantibai's or Harishchandra Yadavaji's doing, it would have appeared normal, being in conformance with the prevailing practice of marrying off girls before pubescence. But, tragically for Rukhmabai, it was done by Sakharam, the man who had outdone Ranade in practising the reform he preached. According to her own testimony 'the chief contracting parties to my marriage' were Sakharam and the mother of the prospective husband. There is no mention of Jayantibai while Harishchandra is said to have been 'only formally consulted as he was my natural father's executor'.[3]

Rukhmabai was categorical about Sakharam's sole responsibility for getting married when she was a child. She was no less categorical about what child marriage made her suffer. In a rare outburst of personal anguish, the characteristically restrained Rukhmabai wrote:

> I am one of those unfortunate Hindu women whose hard lot it is to suffer the unnameable miseries entailed by the custom of early marriage. This wicked practice has destroyed the happiness of my life. It comes between myself and that I prize above all others – study and mental cultivation. Without the least fault of mine, I am doomed to seclusion. Every aspiration of mine, to rise above my ignorant sisters, is looked down upon with suspicion and is interpreted in the most uncharitable manner.[4]

Early marriage was a curse. Getting married to Dadaji, the man chosen by Sakharam, was a greater curse. For, whatever dictated the choice, Rukhmabai's well-being certainly did not. The man was a frail, weak-willed nineteen-year-old good-for-nothing school drop-out, an incorrigible idler from an undistinguished and poor family. Called Dadaji Bhikaji, the man had nothing to commend him in the marriage market. Yet, Dr Sakharam Arjun anointed him his son-in-law.

The mystery of Sakharam's choice is deepened by Rukhmabai's further testimony that Dadaji's mother 'had for years importuned my mother and grandfather to marry me to one of her sons'. Failing to persuade those two, she started pleading with Sakharam for Dadaji. And succeeded.

We must anticipate events to understand how that happened. While hearing the case that involved this unlikeliest of couples, Sir Charles Sargent, the Chief Justice of the Bombay High Court, was intrigued as to how 'this very attractive lady' got 'married to such a man'. The mystery was unveiled for him by Latham, Rukhmabai's astute counsel, from whom little of the case was hidden. In choosing Dadaji, Latham explained, Sakharam had 'acted rather in the interests of his own family than that of the girl'.[5] What Latham told the Chief Justice discreetly was loudly announced in public by a former student of Sakharam, Dr K. R. Kirtikar. Rukhmabai's ruin, said Kirtikar, was plotted by 'her new father … in order to retain her property in his house'.[6]

This is how it transpired. Before Sakharam married the widowed Jayantibai, the substantial property her first husband, Janardan Pandurang, had willed to her was transferred to Rukhmabai. This was done to pre-empt any claims Janardan's kin might make to his property following Jayantibai's remarriage. This necessity arose, ironically, on account of the Hindu Widows Remarriage Act (1856), the very enactment that had entitled Hindu widows to remarry. While entitling widows to do so, the Act had led to conflicting judicial decisions about the remarrying widow's entitlement to her deceased husband's property. The Bombay High Court had interpreted the

Act to deny unprejudiced inheritance to a remarrying widow even if she belonged, like Jayantibai did, to a community that customarily permitted widows to marry again. Belonging to Bombay, Jayantibai and Sakharam had to effect the transfer, or else risk the property being claimed by some covetous relative of Janardan Pandurang's.

This meant that once Rukhmabai was married, the property would go to her husband's family. Sakharam's selection of Dadaji was designed to pre-empt that.

Dadaji was distantly related to Sakharam. A poor idler cousin was unlikely to stand up to an affluent and powerful father-in-law. As a further safeguard, Sakharam also arranged with Dadaji's mother that her son would be a *ghar jamaai*, that is, stay with his in-laws. So, following this arrangement, would the property of Rukhmabai's biological father. Except for this dubious advantage, there was nothing to justify the arrangement. Indeed, the *ghar jamaai* scheme was, *ab initio*, suspect. Dadaji, Sakharam knew, was not 'a good man.' In maintaining that being a *ghar jamaai* and going back to school would make Dadaji a good man, Sakharam was at best dissembling. But for property, he could easily have found Rukhmabai a decent match in the first instance. It is worth noting that in her feminist Marathi text, *Stree-Purush Tulana* (1882), Tarabai Shinde had severely criticized the practice of *ghar jamaai*.[7] The practice, she argued, necessarily involved a husband whose position was inferior to his wife's, and that was a recipe for marital complications and unhappiness.

Rukhmabai herself suspected nothing duplicitous about this marital arrangement – not publicly in any case. We do not know if she said anything to Latham in defence of Sakharam. But she rubbished Kirtikar's charge, calling it a 'base suggestion made by an irresponsible party'. Savaging him, she wrote:

… when I recollect that the writer of the declamation, which bristles
with abuse of my dear father, is the same individual who, whilst

studying at College only a few years back, was dependent on the good-will of my father who was then alive. Witness these quotations from the writer's own letters addressed to Dr Sakharam Arjun: 'You have laid me under further obligation for which recompense at my hands is next to impossible, but you will find me attached to you henceforth as a grateful friend ... I feel it deeply that my connection with you has been a continuous source of gain to me, and those near and dear to me.'[8]

Rukhmabai sought to clinch the argument by pointing out that Sakharam was too wealthy to eye her paltry property. He had, she added, left each of his children from Jayantibai 'better provided for than myself'. But, then, avarice bears no necessary correlation to penury or plenty. Base considerations can cloud the purest minds.

Property threw Rukhmabai into a dangerous domestic trap. She had no idea what was happening – being done – to her. Let alone her – a child – even Sakharam did not know that his little manipulation would return to hit hard. The hardest hit would be Rukhmabai. Property would get her married to Dadaji. Which would mean that many of the miseries she traced to marriage were rooted in property. Without the lure of her property, Narayan Dhurmaji would have never invested in an expensive lawsuit and instigated Dadaji to drag Rukhmabai into the courtroom. Left to himself, the moneyless Dadaji would have had no option but to give up on her and take another wife, which is what he eventually did. Not for nothing had Justice Hannen, an authority on the subject, identified property as the real cause behind suits for the restitution of conjugal rights.

Sakharam had shown his mettle as a reformer in the matter of his own marriage with Jayantibai. He could have done the same for Rukhmabai. Besides, he had before him the example of his father-in-law, Harishchandra Yadavaji. Harishchandra had waited for his daughter to be thirteen before solemnizing her marriage. He had, besides, done that more than a decade earlier when the hold of organized orthodoxy was stronger. To complete the contrast, Harishchandra had found for his daughter an educated, well-off husband, not a pathetic school drop-out. What the orthodox father-in-law did could not have been impossible for the reformer son-in-law.

Except that there was property. At her age, and with her eminent marriage-worthiness, Rukhmabai faced no risk of lifelong spinsterhood in the event of not being married to Dadaji. But there was a real risk of Dadaji and his mother not waiting indefinitely to obtain Rukhmabai. The mother might even have dropped a discreet hint to that effect in the course of importuning Sakharam. If Dadaji was gone, the search for another poor cousin and pliant *ghar jamaai* was likely to be a wild goose chase. It was therefore property, not Sakharam's lapse as a reformer, that precipitated Rukhmabai's marriage.

Sad as this story is, it is amusing to see Dadaji's narration of it. After describing at length the central role of property, he maintained in his 'Exposition':

> I trust that the facts of the case which I have now given will render it quite evident that that scrupulous gentleman, Mr Harichand Jadowji, has alone caused this family rupture, and that a question of property has been represented to the public as a question of Hindu marriage. Can astute jugglery be carried further than this? If the name Harichandra is substituted for the name Rakhmabai in this case, its realities will be better understood but its poetry will be gone.

He concluded:

> If this will [Janardan Pandurang's] and this property had had no existence, there would have been no case of *Dadaji vs. Rakhmabai,*

and there would have been no separation between myself and my lawful wife.

Dadaji was too involved to realize that had this property had no existence, he would not have had Rukhmabai as his lawful wife.

To leave property and return to the miseries of marriage proper, they were many and they made themselves known at different points in time. The earliest to surface was the abrupt termination of Rukhmabai's schooling. This was a cruel blow for a girl who, to quote her, had 'a great passion for studies'. The precocious dreams of a life of service she had started dreaming lay shattered. Matured beyond her years by adversity, she noticed with helpless fury the irony of being removed from school precisely when Dadaji was being forced to resume his education. Education was necessary for her husband to become a good man, not for her to be a good woman!

Yet again Sakharam baffles. He, the champion of higher education for women, pleaded helplessness. He had to submit, he said, to Dadaji's family. They demanded that their daughter-in-law be taken out of school forthwith. It strains credulity that the man who could demand that Dadaji would be a *ghar jamaai* and start going to school again, could not prevail upon the other party to let her schooling continue after marriage. He was not the kind who would give in on matters he felt strongly about. Thus, when Rukhmabai reached puberty six months after her marriage and custom required that she undergo *garbhadhan* – consummation of marriage – Sakharam put his foot down. Not only did he defer *garbhadhan* when it was due, he continued to defer it indefinitely.

Assuming, however, that there were pressures Sakharam could not surmount, he could at least have spared a little time to personally instruct his aspiring daughter. Else he could have got her a lady tutor. There was no dearth of European ladies in Bombay who would have happily accepted the assignment. And Sakharam, known as the

'Lord', was a rich man. A lady tutor was, finally, appointed. But that was after the 'Lord' was dead and Jayantibai had got their eldest son married. The tutor was meant to teach the son's wife, a minor, and the twentysomething Rukhmabai to converse in English.

The enormity of Sakharam's unconcern for his stepdaughter's education comes out when compared with Ranade's dedication to educating his illiterate child-wife, Ramabai. Ranade did this in the face of persistent ridicule and opposition from his family and community. His wife, thanks to his efforts, rose to be a pioneer of women's education.

There are other illustrious exceptions – such as Jotiba Phule who transformed his illiterate wife, Savitri, into his own equal – to show that those who had the will acted in the face of entrenched conservativism. One such individual lived in Sakharam's own neighbourhood, Girgaum. This was Dr Atmaram Pandurang (1823–98).

Fellow professionals, Sakharam and Atmaram were collaborators in a number of public causes. They were the only Indians who were among the founding members of the Bombay Natural History Society. They were also, both of them, members of the Bombay Medical and Physical Society. As Indian doctors operating within a system dominated by Western doctors and Western medicine, they sought to get proper recognition for traditional systems of medication, and objected to systemic discrimination against Indian vis-à-vis British doctors in India. When Atmaram founded the Prarthana Samaj, Sakharam donated money for its 'Prarthana Mandir' and delivered some of its weekly lectures for women.

But there was also between them a contrast which Rukhmabai would have acutely felt. Atmaram afforded all his children the best possible education without discriminating between his five sons and three daughters. He sent his second daughter, Annapoorna, to England for three years when she was seventeen, and his youngest daughter, Manak, to Bombay's Grant Medical College and to Edinburgh for further medical training.

Atmaram, unlike Sakharam, also saved his children from early marriage. He even encouraged them to mix with the opposite sex and marry for love. To provide a particularly striking example, he had seventeen-year-old Rabindranath Tagore stay in his house for two months and learn English conversation from twenty-year-old Annapoorna who was just back from England. It is believed that on discovering that the young couple had developed mutual attraction, Atmaram journeyed with Annapoorna to Calcutta, but the match was unacceptable to Rabindranath's father, Devendranath Tagore.

Even if apocryphal, the storied journey to Calcutta is plausible. It describes the person Atmaram was. For, only two years later, he was blessing Annapoorna as she married Harold Littledale, an Irishman with whom she had fallen in love. Atmaram was equally accepting when Manak presented him with a Parsi son-in-law, barrister Dorab Nausserwanji Bahadurji. Happy to have a cosmopolitan family – an embodiment of the ancient motto of *vasudhaiva kutumbakam* – he also welcomed into it two English daughters-in-law. The same catholicity of vision enabled him to remain a fond father to a daughter – Annapoorna – and two sons even after they converted to Christianity.

Tragically for Rukhmabai, Sakharam failed to be the model guardian a celebrated social reformer should have been. If only Sakharam were to her what Atmaram was to his children, she would have wistfully thought.

Yet, descriptions of Sakharam's guardianship of Rukhmabai have been unreservedly celebratory. He is credited with making Rukhmabai the confident, cultured, prepossessing person she was. He is even seen as the man who 'encouraged' her 'to pursue medical studies'.[9] In a recent reiteration of this celebratory narrative, Kavitha Rao writes:

... even Dr Sakharam was not powerful enough to defy Hindu custom and stop Rukhmabai being married off as a child ... Dr Sakharam was uncomfortable with the marriage. Later, he would participate in efforts to reform Hindu customs, and would speak passionately in favour of separating Hindu law from Hindu custom. Dr Sakharam would also go on to recommend that young children betrothed in marriage should have the chance to 'ratify' the marriage once older. This was a radical thought for the time, and one can see how Rukhmabai might have idolised this unusual, charismatic man.[10]

But, it may be argued, Rukhmabai did idolize Sakharam. Whatever little she wrote about her life was during the pendency of her historic case. That small body of writing shows Rukhmabai portraying Sakharam as a caring, loving and sympathetic father. Read closely, the same body of work also betrays a contrary undercurrent which corroborates the foregoing facts-based unfavourable portrayal of Sakharam. The truth is that more than showing what he actually did for her, Rukhmabai's idolizing of Sakharam shows the father she – an orphan – wanted to possess.

Girl Rukhmabai was not married long when she was forced through a horrifying experience. Growing up turned into a nightmare, and fear of men entered into her being forever. A decade later she would say in a letter that she had 'a great disgust for married life' and trace the disgust back to her 'childhood'.[11] She mentions no specific details, and it is possible that the disgust grew from what she saw of conjugality as a child. But her intensity in expressing the disgust suggests something personal and traumatic. The following experience very likely is what that was.

Dadaji's mother, having pulled off her little miracle, was happy that, as Sakharam's *ghar jamaai*, her rotten son would become a good man. But she died four months later and the son walked out on his planned transformation. He succumbed to the lure of an indolent and indulgent life with his maternal uncle, Narayan Dhurmaji.

Narayan was an embodiment of the villainous *mama* – maternal uncle – immortalized through the figure of Shakuni in the *Mahabharata*. Untouched by human decency and filled with petty cunning, Narayan was a middling contractor of some means. Sheltering his nephew in defiance of his deceased sister's plan was part of Narayan's own crafty counter-plan. He would stoke his nephew's wayward ways, occasionally employ and pay him for petty odd jobs, and keep advancing him loans. Narayan's design was to reduce him into a parasite so that whenever Rukhmabai joined her husband, she would come to Narayan's house. And with her would come her property – the property of a spineless indebted dependent's wife.

Narayan was also an impudent lech. Cheap everyday escapades apart, he had picked up from a lime factory a nineteen-year-old labourer named Chinnama – Chinoo – as his mistress. That was common practice. What was uncommon was Narayan's brazenness in bringing the mistress home and foisting her on his family. We can only imagine the effect it would have had on Narayan's children. But we know for certain what it did to his poor wife. Unable to bear the ordeal, she resolved to liberate herself – 'to avoid the tyranny' of the mistress, as Rukhmabai put it – and jumped into the family well.

The incident was damning. Even more damning was Narayan's nonchalance about it. At the centre of a defamation suit which this man filed, and lost, against Rukhmabai, her grandfather and Grattan Geary, the editor of the *Bombay Gazette*, was Rukhamabai's public disclosure of the liaison. Geary was dragged into the case for publishing Rukhmabai's impugned statement. He chose to defend himself in the magistrate's court. The following excerpt from Geary's cross-examination of Narayan says it all:

Geary: You know your wife jumped into a well.

Witness: I heard so.

Geary: Was it for the purpose of killing herself?

Witness: I do not know. I cannot say.

Geary: Did she jump into the well to take a bath?

Witness: It might be so. She was at the time wrong in her head. She had been suffering from fever, and I cannot say for what reason she went into the well.

Geary: Did not the neighbours tell you she went in to kill herself?

Witness: No.

Geary: Who took her out?

Witness: Some men.

Geary: Did you ask the men how she got in?

Witness: Perhaps, I did. I had asked Ardesheer on my return, and I then heard she had fallen into the well.

Geary: What were their names?

Witness: The men who took her out were not present when I returned. I do not know their names.

Geary: Did not anyone tell you that your wife had told these men she had jumped into the well on account of this woman [Chinnama]?

Witness: No.

Geary: Do you know that Rukhmabai said so?

Witness: No, I do not know.[12]

Rukhmabai called this man 'evil-minded'. It was to live in his house that Dadaji had walked out of Sakharam's. During the first year of her marriage, Rukhmabai went there a few times. One day she resolved never to go there again. The resolve and its severe observance is all we know for a fact. Even when, as late as 1884, she was persuaded to consider cohabitation with Dadaji, she was adamant that she would not go to him in Narayan's house.

During her visits there in the first year of her marriage, she may have sensed something eerie in that house. But that could not have warranted the resolve to never enter that house. Something more sinister had to happen to occasion the resolve.

As lecherous as he was covetous, Narayan desired not only the property of his dependent nephew's wife but also her body. She was visiting his house when one night he found his chance and made advances to her. That is when, shaken and traumatized, she resolved to never return there.

What concupiscent Narayan did was nothing unheard of. Sexual abuse by unscrupulous family elders of their young wards' wives was rampant. These elders even used the practice of early marriage to their advantage by getting the family's young boys wedded to girls older than them. Disparity of age saved the elders the agony of waiting for the new brides' pubescence; they would be ready for copulation.

Another pointer to that night's lecherous advance by Narayan lies buried in Rukhmabai's letter to the *Times of India* on the evil of early marriage. A palpable urgency comes into the letter when she discusses the evil of girls being married to boys younger than them. The matter-of-fact tone of suggesting ways to eradicate early marriage suddenly becomes imperative: 'Under no circumstances shall the wife be older than the husband.'[13] Having been vulnerable even as the wife of an adult, Rukhmabai worried that older girls picked for marriage to minor boys were sitting ducks for the family's male prowlers.

However, the decisive evidence on this – if we can have the imagination to see it as evidence – comes from a novelist. In her fictional portrayal of Rukhmabai's life, *Mala He Lagna Manya Nahi*, Sarojini Sharangpani describes the incident in vivid detail:

Lost in her thoughts, Rukhmi was sitting in the room, shedding tears, unable to decide anything. Just then, pushing the door quietly, someone came in. He moved towards her. A ray of light suddenly entered the dark of the room. Rukhmi looked up and found Narayan looming over her. This man here at this time! She got up and asked in a subdued voice: 'What are you looking for? I will find it for you.'

'There is nothing to find. It is with you.' Narayan laughed. Rukhmi found that laughter bizarre. She took two quick steps and was instantly out of the room. She was in no mental state to explain why she did that. She couldn't say anything. She was filled with fear, and her heartbeat shot up suddenly.

Narayan left immediately after Rukhmi came out of the room. He obviously had nothing to do there. Why then, Rukhmi wondered, did he come in and why did he take off just like that? He had looked at Rukhmi while leaving. It was a sinister lustful look.[14]

Barring proven exceptions, that one look would henceforth define men for Rukhmabai.

The foregoing account might create the impression of cheer coming to Rukhmabai during the brief interregnum between her entry into Sakharam's family and her marriage. That is not what exactly happened. Of course, life in this family was not like it was in her maternal grandfather's family. Many good things would happen here. Indeed, Rukhmabai would become here the woman she was. But cheer eluded her here too. The sad, introverted girl continued to be sad and introverted. Hers was a uniformly cheerless growing up.

Let us begin with a rare account we have of Rukhmabai's domestic routine. Nora Scott writes in her *Indian Journal*:

She leads a busy life, not only because she studies, but she does a great deal in the house. She takes entire charge of the little girl and younger boy, washing and dressing them and having them with her constantly. Her grandmother cooks for the family, and her mother is not strong, but if the grandmother is away, or ill, then Miss Sakharam does the cooking.[15]

Rukhmabai never complained of this burden. But she decried the way daughters-in-law were routinely treated as worse than servants:

She must get up early and go to bed late. Must work with the servants (I do not say like the servants, for they have the option of refusing to work, which she has not).[16]

There was, of course, a qualitative difference between a daughter engaged in household work and a daughter-in-law subjected to the same under a callous mother-in-law. Yet, this account matches Nora Scott's description of Rukhmabai's hard, dreary life. What needs to be added is that the burden Rukhmabai bore day and night was heavier than appears in Scott's description. The 'little girl and younger boy' whose 'entire charge' rested on Rukhmabai, and whom she had 'with her constantly,' were her half-siblings. They were five, not just two. Similarly, Scott's description of Jayantibai as 'not strong' hides in it a never-ending remorseless pressure on young Rukhmabai's time and energy.

Sakharam lived but twelve years with Jayantibai. They produced five children. There was also a sixth pregnancy which ended in a still birth towards the end of 1884. That made it one pregnancy every two years. As a celebrated physician concerned with issues of social reform, especially the amelioration of women in his society, Sakharam had taken it upon himself to write popular books in Marathi on issues of physical and moral well-being. One of these books – *Vivah Vigyan* – was on marriage, and another – *Garbhavidya va Prasutikaran* – on pregnancy and childhood. Though birth control was yet to become a public issue, Sakharam would have known about the current advances in the field. One may wonder if he never thought of doing something to protect his young and increasingly frail wife from frequent pregnancies. Or was it that he tried and did not succeed?

It was Jayantibai's pregnancies that made her 'not strong' and took her away from household chores for extended periods. Per force, young Rukhmabai and her step-grandmother had to shoulder between them an increasing share of the household work, including the care of the growing number of babies.

Rukhmabai's first half-sibling was born before she was ten. That made her a 'little mother' and the half-siblings who followed kept her in the role. She always had one or two very young ones whose urgent demands could come any time of the day and night. She had no time she could call her own. She was obliged to carry one or more of the young ones along even on her formal social visits. Thus, when she first called on Nora Scott, Rukhmabai was accompanied by 'her two little brothers and little sister'. The second time, which was for a party, she was accompanied by four siblings. As Scott wrote in her *Journal*:

Then Rukmabai came with her two little brothers and sisters; her father continuing a little better she had been able to come. It must have been a long work for her to get all these children into such gala attire – for I know she has scarcely any help now in her care of the children, when her mother is engaged entirely in nursing Dr Sakharam. The little girl … whom I had last seen in a little white nightgown, now appeared in a flowered silk jacket and long skirt reaching to her feet. The younger boy, of two, who was in a simpler costume at my last interview – as then he had nothing on whatsoever – was resplendent in a peach-coloured silk suit and a jacket pointed at the back and edged with gold braid, trousers to match, and a jaunty cap embroidered in gold and silver. The boy of four, whose bare legs had before attracted the attention of Bracken (the dog), appeared in a rich brown satin costume, and very handsome the little fellow looked with his splendid black eyes. I could not do much to amuse the children, having the ladies to attend to, but they seemed quite happy.[17]

Left to herself, Rukhmabai would rather have gone alone on such occasions. But there was little she could do about it. Going out just for fun and enjoyment was not for her.

Nora Scott has also described a particularly haunting incident. It happened on 24 June 1884 by when all of Rukhmabai's half-siblings had been born. She writes:

> Yesterday the Hindu lady I had met at Miss Pechey's came to spend the afternoon with me. She brought her two little brothers and little sister … They arrived at about a quarter to five … I asked the children if they would like to go out and play in the garden, and Nellie brought out the battledores and shuttlecocks for them. They gazed in astonishment when we showed them how to play, but had no notion of playing themselves. Miss Sakharam said 'they would like very much to go out in the garden but,' she added, 'our children never play, you know.' [18]

The words 'our children never play' hit us. They hit Scott, too. Children who *never* play, in what does their being children lie? This is what she felt:

> If the old saying is true 'All work and no play makes Jack a dull boy,' I think 'no work and no play' either, must make him still duller, and that is what the children's lives here seem to me often to be. They have no good games, and they seem to be turned into little men and little women too soon. Miss Sakharam told me that the early marriage stops the girls' education altogether at 10 or 11 years of age. [19]

Scott bemoaned the premature demise of childhood in India. She may as well have added that while Indian children were precociously turned into little men and little women, female children were turned into little women sooner than were male children into little men.

'Our children never play' is clearly an overstatement. Maybe Rukhmabai herself meant it to be taken with a pinch of salt. But it is literally true for her. Neither at Harishchandra's nor at Sakharam's did she ever play. She was never a child. She had not known what it was to be pampered, spoiled and indulged. Nor innocent, aimless fun either. She was busy mothering when she could have been a child.

Rukhmabai never complained about the heavy burden of domestic chores. But there was an aspect of it that upset her badly. Refusing to let her life be ruined by the denial of schooling, she resolved to be an autodidact. This is how she went about it:

> I began to learn English at home after leaving school. I used to ask a number of pronunciations and meanings of English words at a time whenever my European friends happened to call. Day by day my love for education and social reform increased, and I continued to pursue my studies as much as I could, but in this country it is very hard for women to study at home.[20]

This little autobiographical fragment cries for close empathetic reading. What she directly reports in it is important. But much more crucial is that of which she leaves the vaguest trace. Thus, the mode of her study at home is plainly reported, but the pain, shame and loneliness of her inner world are so camouflaged as to be nearly unrecognizable. Sanity demanded that she unburden herself of some of that pain, shame and loneliness, but doing that threatened greater pain and shame. She could not possibly tell the wide world that she had no one at home to sympathize with her passion for education, not even her mother or her affluent social reformer father. She came up with an effective strategy. She would weave her personal pain deceptively into larger observations about society. Hidden in her plaint about study at home being 'very hard' for women 'in this country' is her secret insufferable pain.

A good deal more lies buried in this fragment. For one, Rukhmabai's indomitable will. She was not exceptional in that her schooling had been discontinued after marriage. But she was so in refusing to remain ignorant and let this blow shatter her dreams. Here, perhaps, is the first intimation of the determination that, a mere eight years later, would blossom into her great resistance.

The fragment also points to Rukhmabai's loneliness in the Sakharam household. The European ladies coming to the house were not the only ones who could have instructed her. The house was frequented also by some of the leading social reformers and scholars of the day. R. G. Bhandarkar, eminent savant with pronounced reformist leanings, was Sakharam's neighbour. His daughter, Shanta, and Rukhmabai were intimate friends. Not one of those luminaries felt moved to help the girl. Rukhmabai was in a sea of learning, and thirsting.

But then, Sakharam, too, did not help. If he had, Rukhmabai would certainly have mentioned him. More so because she was always at pains to present him as a wonderful father. Her silence is therefore telling. It is voiced by Kirtikar. Recalling his student days, when he was part of the family, he swore that he never saw Sakharam take any part in educating Rukhmabai. The home was an emotional wilderness.

Of that wilderness she never spoke. The only way to get a feel of it – of the pervasive sadness of her life – is to dig into her melancholy generalizations, of which she has left behind more than the one discussed above.

The same strategy of revealing while concealing is followed in this next example. Here the personal brims over instead of being buried deep within. Rukhmabai was persuaded that no social reform was possible without legislation by the government. But legislation was in those days bitterly opposed on the ground that genuine reform required public awakening and education, not legislation by foreign rulers. The argument was plausible and, for a variety of reasons, enjoyed wide acceptance. Rukhmabai tore into its proponents and believers:

> Can any of these gentlemen honestly tell us what enlightenment they have introduced, or even tried to introduce? If, Sir, educated men like these, who fully admit the existence of the evils, have neither the pluck nor the strong sense of duty to fight them, need we wonder at the indifference of the uneducated masses? In a society where the educated, or the 'upper ten' are indifferent and the uneducated ignorant, is it rash to invoke Government aid for the redress of these crying grievances?[21]

This is polemical writing at its most disturbing. It lays bare the dissembling and bad faith of social reformers, and voices the chagrin of the women victims of their chicanery.

It is even more disturbing as an exercise in autobiographical writing. Here, too, Rukhmabai gives vent to an agony that she has long nursed within her. There is nothing explicitly personal in it. No examples are given nor any names cited in her collective castigation of the 'upper ten'. Also, Rukhmabai, the dutiful daughter, never tired of praising Sakharam as an 'unusually kind stepfather'. She never accused him of showing 'neither the pluck nor the strong sense of duty' to do his duty as a reformist father. Yet, Sakharam's presence among the anonymous 'upper ten' is loud and clear.

Rukhmabai, it is noteworthy, wrote this castigation just two months after Sakharam's death, an event that had left her broken and alone. In his death, she had lost her strongest supporter in the ugly legal battle. Even in the hour of his death her repressed pain came out. It was, indeed, unbearable.

Rukhmabai's love and gratitude for Sakharam was not fake. She told the truth when she said: 'He protected and loved me as his own child throughout his life.'[22] But that was not her whole truth. The pain and hurt she so wrestled to hide was as much part of that truth.

This was the kind of complex truth that characterizes all intimate familial relationships; and into it were thrown the aggravating difficulties of a step-relationship. Most complex vis-à-vis Sakharam, her relationship with Harishchandra and Jayantibai, too, was complex. There was also something pathetic about all her three guardians. Its most moving manifestation comes in the lengths to which she went to protect them against all criticism, foul or fair.

Rukhmabai was too intelligent and human to never suspect that Sakharam had not been entirely fair to her. But, whether it was her property, marriage or education, she never let out a word against him. She rather struggled to excise the gnawing doubts and thoughts from her consciousness, and consigned them to the inaccessible secrecy of her heart. That struggle could even lead her to believe – or say – that Sakharam 'looked to my education'. And credit him for delaying her marriage: 'I was married at the age of 11 years (an age rather beyond the limit of the fixed marriageable age in girls) ...'

Harishchandra and Jayantibai also she defended fiercely. For long neither the mother nor the grandfather understood Rukhmabai's horror of having to live with Dadaji. Even when Sakharam backed her resolve to wash her hands of Dadaji, both Harishchandra and Jayantibai persisted in their efforts to make the marriage work. It was only after Sakharam died and she was left all alone that they gave in to her importunities to stand by her. Yet, she never spoke a word about the stress and uncertainty caused by her mother and grandfather.

Except that defending them did not quite drive her to points that bordered on untruth. She felt obliged, for example, to defend them when Dadaji wrote:

In 1884 I asked that my wife might be allowed to come and live with me ... To my surprise this request was the signal for the open hostility, not of my wife, Rakhmabai, be it remembered, but of her mother, Jaentibai, and her grandfather, Mr Harichandra Jadowji, who feared that if Rakhmabai came to live with me, she would assert her right to the property of her deceased father, the late Mr Junardhun Pandurang, and which property is of the estimated value of upwards of Rs.25,000 ... My mother-in-law, Jaentibai, and her father, Harichandra Jadowji, are now in the enjoyment of the said property ... There is property in this case, and also a mother-in-law, both very good things in their way, but beyond these two great social factors there is nothing special, and absolutely nothing Hindu, in it.[23]

Rukhmabai rubbished the charge, saying:

... my mother inherits from my father, Dr Sakharam, money over and above what I inherited from my natural father ... each of her other children is better provided for than myself ... Mr Hurichand Yadowjee is a well-to-do man, whose long and faithful service has been rewarded by Government with a special title and a special personal allowance in addition to his pension ...

Need I say that all these insinuations with regard to property are entirely false and made to divert the public mind from the real issue in the matter?[24]

Rukhmabai was right. Besides, Jayantibai and Harishchandra were the ones who had tried till the last moment to make the doomed marriage work. Clearly, Dadaji's charge against them was intended to reduce Rukhmabai's epochal fight for women's freedom and dignity to a petty property dispute. She also added:

> My mother inherited the property absolutely by the will of my father, and that I received it is purely due to her affection for me. Before marrying the late Dr Sakharam Arjun, she could have, if she had wished, claimed and disposed of it herself.[25]

Rukhmabai was right. It was, indeed, possible for Jayantibai to dispose of the property before marrying Sakharam. But she transferred it to her daughter. Whatever suspicions arise on account of property relate to Sakharam. And these arose from his choice of Dadaji as Rukhmabai's husband. There is nothing to implicate Jayantibai or Harishchandra Yadavaji.

Rukhmabai was too young to understand anything about property when it was transferred to her. Later on, from bits of conversations within the family, she got a vague sense of some property which her mother, naturally out of love, had given to her. It was during the litigation, when charges and counter-charges were flying around, that a niggling suspicion got into her that there could be more to the transfer of property. Then came in open court her own lawyer's charge that Sakharam had not acted in her interest. No more could Rukhmabai resist being undeceived.

It was a painful undeception. It confronted Rukhmabai with the ugly truth that the ingrate Kirtikar was right about Sakharam in the matter of property. She might still persist in her public defence of the departed stepfather, but that would not heal her inner wounds.

The undeception cost Rukhmabai her innocence. She had come of age. The iron had entered her soul.

It must be said that in his heart of hearts Sakharam had possibly begun to feel guilty at least about the end of Rukhmabai's schooling. That redounds to his credit. What does not is the fact that he nonetheless sought to exonerate himself. Showing us the person he was, he claimed:

> We are also painfully aware that our efforts in eradicating old evils and in sowing new blessings; our attempts at reform, social and religious, which we believe to be fraught with immense good for generations to come, are baffled and foiled by opposition encountered, not on the public platform or the native press, but in the bosom of our own families. How many of our vaunted reformers have had to eat their own words to meekly practise in private what they eloquently denounced in public because their wives and mothers, sisters and cousins proved too strong for them.[26]

The foregoing is the unremembered of Rukhmabai's early life. Let us now turn to that which is remembered and celebrated. Both true, the unremembered and the remembered together show that life for Rukhmabai in Sakharam's house was at the same time constraining and liberating.

A good deal of what Rukhmabai underwent during those unhappy years, we have seen, was a function of the times she was born and brought up in. We have also seen that the reality of Sakharam does not quite square with Rukhmabai's image of him as an 'unusually kind stepfather'. Now we shall see that he was also the kind of father she believed him to be. She was, undoubtedly, lucky to have come under his guardianship. She may not have got the facilities a girl intent on educating herself deserved. Nonetheless, if she grew to be a cultivated and aware person, it was largely on account of being in that household. There she did not have to study on the sly. Nor did seeking education bring upon her, as it typically did upon Ramabai Ranade, the family's scorn and anger.

Further, it was the Sakharam household that offered her the privilege of the European lady visitors who kindly turned into her informal tutors. In fact, her interaction with those European ladies was not confined to home. Sakharam encouraged young Rukhmabai to go out and cultivate her contacts with them. This also brought the additional advantage that her study was not limited within the short intervals stolen out of never-ending domestic duties. Especially helpful in this respect were her regular visits to Bombay's Christian mission houses and their libraries. The one she frequented the most was the American Mission House during the time of the much-loved missionary couple, Mr and Mrs Hume.

Indeed, breathing the liberal atmosphere of Sakharam's house was an inspiration to evolve into a cultured person. For one, the sight of her famous stepfather poring over books, journals and newspapers in his impressive study, or writing away, presented the impressionable girl with a model for emulation. She would, given a half-chance, go into that wondrous space and discover bits of its treasures. No less inspiring was to see among the visitors to the house some of the finest minds of the day and eavesdrop on their wide-ranging conversations. She would write later:

> ... constant association with the people who had tried to devote their lives to the social reform of India, and by the aid of the little education which I had been able to gain, I began seriously to consider the former and present condition of our Hindu women, and wished to do something, if in my power, to ameliorate our present sufferings.[27]

Growing up in the Sakharam household was a privilege her coevals could at best have envied. One of her great blessings was escaping the physical–mental torture of routine beatings that marked an average Indian female's entire life. Something of that harrowing reality – not yet consigned to the past – can be imagined by recalling the life of an illustrious contemporary of Rukhmabai, Anandibai Joshee (1865–87).

Anandibai was the first Indian woman to leave the Indian shores and return as a qualified doctor. She was just twenty-one when, in March 1886, she became a doctor from the Women's Medical College of Pennsylvania, the first medical college for women in the world. The following year, before she could take up her assignment in Kolhapur, she was dead. Much in Anandibai's wasted life is heart-rending; the most heart-rending are the beatings she was subjected to. Pre-marriage the tormentor was her mother; then the function was taken up by her husband. In a letter from the USA in 1884, Anandibai told her husband:

> My mother … never spoke to me affectionately. When she punished me, she was wont to use not just a small rope or thong, but always stones, sticks and live charcoal. Fortunately, my body does not bear any scars, and her severe beating did not leave me maimed, crippled or deformed. By the grace of God, my limbs survived intact! But oh! the sheer agony of those memories! … Unfortunate indeed is the child which has missed a happy childhood.[28]

Anandibai's husband was Gopal Vinayak Joshee. Gopal, a widower, was twenty-nine and Anandibai barely nine when they were married. In many ways an extraordinary man, Gopal was way ahead even of Ranade in promoting his wife's education. Initially, like Ranade, he arranged for his wife's schooling, and then, surpassing his famous compatriot, arranged to send her to the USA for medical education. But even this husband did not bring to an end Anandibai's ordeal. She writes in the same letter:

> It is not at all my intention to distress your dear heart or to cause a

rift in our love by raking up old memories ... It is very difficult to decide whether your treatment of me was good or bad. If you ask me, I would answer that it was both. It seems to have been right in view of its ultimate goal; but, in all fairness, one is compelled to admit that it was wrong, considering its possible effects on a child's mind. Hitting me with broken pieces of wood at the tender age of ten, flinging chairs and books at me and threatening to leave me when I was twelve, and inflicting other strange punishments on me when I was fourteen – all these were too severe for the age, body and mind at each respective stage ... If I had left you at that immature age, as you kept on suggesting, what would have happened? I would have been lost. (And any number of girls have left their homes because of harassment from mothers-in-law and husbands.) I did not do so because I was afraid that my ill-considered behaviour would tarnish my father's honour ... And I begged you not to spare me, but to kill me. In our society, for centuries there has been no legal restraint between husbands and wives, and if it exists, it works against women! Such being the case, I had no recourse but to allow you to hit me with chairs and bear it with equanimity. A Hindu woman has no right to utter a word or to advise her husband. On the contrary, she has a right to allow her husband to do what he wishes and to keep quiet ... I was born to endure all that.[29]

No less disturbing is the following sequence in Anandibai's biography by Caroline Healey Dall, an American, which came out within a year of Anandibai's premature death:

In a letter written by Gopal to one of his friends in this country, during the distracted days that followed his wife's death in Poona, he says, 'I wonder if she would not be living still, if I had never gone to America.'

Strange that he should have written this, and stranger still would he have deemed it, had he known that the one thought that rang through my brain as we sat together day after day in Philadelphia was this: 'He will make life impossible for her.'[30]

It is possible that the brutality inflicted on Anandibai was greater than what girls and women in her society were subjected to as a matter of course. But neither that brutality nor the trauma it produced was atypical. Sakharam protected Rukhmabai from both.

He also protected her from another trauma. He did not permit, as we have seen above, the *garbhadhan* ceremony following her pubescence six months after her marriage. If permitted, that would have forced Rukhmabai into sexual intercourse with her nineteen-year-old husband before she had turned twelve. Also, possibly, into early motherhood, as frequently happened then, and had happened to her own mother.

The nightmare of consummation for the helpless girl-wife must be visualized in concrete human terms. Let us turn again to Anandibai's life. This time to her biography by an Indian admirer, Kashibai Kanitkar (1861–1948), which, too, like the biography by Dall, came out in the year following Anandibai's death. A contemporary of Anandibai, and one of the makers of early modern Marathi literature, Kashibai was actively involved in women's movements for reform. Right in the beginning of the biography, Kashibai says that Anandibai was so full of strange fears that for days she just refused to enter her husband's bedroom. She believed that there was a tiger in that room. Like Anandibai, Kashibai, too, was married when she was nine. It is possible that the fears of Anandibai that she described were her fears too.

All girl-wives underwent that torment, even if not all imagined tigers. Some might have visualized other scary images, while many others might have straightaway seen the husband as the tormentor. The torment was lifelong. In many aggravated cases, it even led to hysteria. And deadened the child-wife to the beauty and ecstasy of sex.

Rukhmabai was fortunate to have escaped that nightmare. But that early close brush with the ugliness of sexual passion was enough to turn her against its rewards. A letter written on 23 June 1886 to Edith Pechey – one of the first women doctors in the United Kingdom and an advocate for women's healthcare, work and education in India – is revealing in this respect. Returning one of the two books Pechey had lent her – F. Marion Crawford's bestselling 1884 novel, *A Roman Singer* – Rukhmabai peremptorily dismissed it: 'I looked it all over just enough to know the purport of the story, which I found contains nothing but *mere love matters*.'[31] Except for a lively friendship with a bright young man in London, she would all her life remain averse to man–woman relations.

We may anticipate later events to conclude this brief assessment of Rukhmabai's gains from being Sakharam's daughter. The enormity of wedding her to Dadaji eventually dawned on Sakharam, and he resolved to stand by her. This particular guilt he could never get over and died with it. Of his end there is the following moving account in Nora Scott's *Journal*:

> It was the one trouble that embittered the good stepfather's last hours – almost his last words to her were on this subject. He blamed himself for not having collected more evidence about the man – he was leaving her alone to fight the case ...[32]

The repentant father's last words to the wronged daughter were: 'You must trust to your friends ... Mrs Scott and Miss Pechey and Mrs Curjel.' Miss Pechey more than justified Sakharam's faith. Of Mrs Curjel we know little beyond her being the wife of a merchant and banking agent. In any case, she was away in Lahore during much of the pendency of Rukhmabai's case. And Nora Scott, who could have done anything for Rukhmabai, was rendered helpless by being a judge's wife:

> But I could hardly show her even sympathy, for directly John [Justice Scott] heard that the case was on his list, he said of course that I must not go to her house, or ask her to come here. Then, poor girl, when she wrote to me asking me to speak to John, I could not even write to her, or see her at Miss Pechey's house, or anywhere else. Miss Pechey had tried to make her understand that no party in a suit must attempt to influence the judge, but it was impossible to make her see it in an English point of view. I am certain she did not mean to do anything the least dishonourable.[33]

Scott, uncharacteristically for an Englishwoman in India, understood Rukhmabai's incomprehension of the 'English point of view'. But we, after nearly two centuries of living with Western jurisprudence, may be tempted to fault Rukhmabai. It is important, therefore, to remember that when she was hauled up before an English judge, the new judicial system had been in operation for just two and a half decades. She had not imbibed the logic of valuing procedure more than the truth of her cause.

Scott understood, felt acutely for her brave 'Hindu friend', and followed the case restlessly from a distance. The moment the verdict came in her friend's favour, Scott sent forth her congratulations and received the following reply:

> Thank you for your kind note. I am so thankful to God that He has heard our prayers and saved me from the perpetual misery, and brought the truth to light at last. – With kind regards, Yours affectionately, Rukhmabai.[34]

Let us return to Sakharam's penitence. Even after he had decided to make amends, there were limits beyond which he could not, being a stepfather, oppose what Rukhmabai's mother and grandfather wished to be done in her case. Sakharam had to be diplomatic, not adamant.

While Rukhmabai blossomed into a refined young woman in the midst of the difficulties and blessings of the Sakharam household, the wishful plan for her husband's transformation collapsed sooner than its worst critics had predicted. Within 'a few months after the marriage', Rukhmabai reported, Dadaji:

> began to neglect his duties, leaving the school, and disobeying my father and grandfather, fell into bad companies. I should rather say the consequence of which was that he fell sick, and was attacked with consumption, confined to his bed for three continuous years, in such a state that he was not expected to live another season. But by God's grace he recovered a little day by day.[35]

In a later account, Rukhmabai was even more forthright:

> He abused my relatives, including my mother, in language which was shameful. He set at defiance the efforts made by my father and grandfather to educate him, and took to ways which a woman's lips cannot utter. Mr Dadaji went through every course of dissipation ...[36]

Dadaji, spurning the great chance his mother had got him, remained a confirmed wastrel. In the meanwhile, Rukhmabai, defying crushing difficulties, engaged herself assiduously in self-cultivation. In their contrasting development lay the near inevitability of her struggle for women's emancipation.

An ironic sociological reversal – deeply tragic for Rukhmabai – also lay in that contrast. Given the bleak state of female education, males who had acquired English education and, as a sequel, a different kind of sensibility, found themselves in varying measure of incompatibility with their wives. Rife with grave consequences, the incompatibility even led to many desertions. Rukhmabai's was a rare instance in which the wife was the superior spouse. But, unlike men burdened with wives unfitted for them, she did not enjoy the luxury of walking out on her spouse. She was expected to submit and suffer in silence.

She was even warned that her defiance – her refusal to submit and suffer – would harm the very women whose champion she claimed to be. For, if she questioned her marriage on the ground that she was married when she was too young to give intelligent consent, she would encourage men to leave their wives at will, arguing that these unfit wives had been forced upon them when they were incapable of consenting to the marriage. This argument was widely believed. As if men were not already deserting their wives at will and with abandon. And needed a Rukhmabai to be shown the way.

It seems that by the time Rukhmabai left for England, the worst was behind her. Her three guardians had done enough to help her get over that which she could have held against them. The most extraordinary of the three, of course, had been Sakharam. His death in the moment of being his persecuted daughter's best friend was truly a shattering loss for her. She, fulfilling a long-orphaned girl's longing for a loving father, had all along been drawn to him. Losing him when they had really come close reinforced the favourable image she had entertained of him.

Rukhmabai's narrative of Sakharam as a caring, loving and sympathetic father gained wide currency and credence in England. It was reproduced, occasionally re-embellished, each time Rukhmabai was written and spoken about. For instance, at one of her first public lectures, in Bristol, the chairperson said of the speaker's stepfather:

> This gentleman practised as a medical man; he appreciated education
> and had Rukhmabai educated, and in course of time she grew up

into a cultivated person, while her obnoxious *fiancé* seems to have descended the social scale.[37]

To sum up the meaning of Sakharam in Rukhmabai's life, it seems reasonable to propose that Rukhmabai, indeed, became Rukhmabai – capable of big things – during her years at Sakharam's. This was as should have been under the guardianship of a person like Sakharam. But this happened not entirely because, but also in spite, of him. More than Sakharam, Rukhmabai's own will and determination made her what she became.

The conflicting claims relating to her birth and marriage may appear trivial today, but they are of critical significance for understanding the marital dispute that would change the course of Rukhmabai's life.

Rukhmabai is believed to have been born on 22 November 1864. For the better part of colonial India, unless proved otherwise, ascribed dates and, even more, years of birth are unreliable. There was in those days no compulsory registration of births and deaths. Nor of marriages. If someone's date and year of birth needed to be provided, say for admission to a school or for filing a suit concerning inheritance or marriage, those dates were suitably fabricated.

Horoscopes can, generally, be relied upon. But they are rarely available. Till not long ago, it was common for individuals to have two dates of birth: the actual and the 'official'. Many such people are still alive. I know of a brother and sister, the age difference between whom, going by their official dates of birth, is six months.

According to the papers submitted before the Bombay High Court on behalf of Rukhmabai, she was eleven at the time of her marriage. As against this, her husband claimed that she was thirteen. However, the rival parties were agreed that the marriage was solemnized in 1876. Given this agreement, Dadaji's claim pushes back Rukhmabai's year of birth to 1863. The same year is also suggested by Justice

Pinhey, the only judge who ruled in favour of Rukhmabai. Delivering his judgment in September 1885, Pinhey described Rukhmabai as an intelligent young woman of twenty-two. But he also said that Rukhmabai was married when she was eleven, which would push back her marriage to 1874, whereas the year of their marriage – 1876 – is the only point on which both she and Dadaji were in agreement.

Rukhmabai and, naturally, her friends and well-wishers stuck to 1865 as the year of her birth. Thus, in her application form for admission to the London School of Medicine for Women, she declared herself to be twenty-four. Considering that the application was submitted on 29 September 1890, two months before she became twenty-five, 1865 emerges as the year of her birth. Similarly, in a memorial submitted to the Government of India in 1887, the Rukhmabai Defence Committee described her as a woman of twenty-two who had been married eleven years back. But then, at the time of her graduation, 1864 was officially given as the year of her birth.

Like with the year of Rukhmabai's birth, we cannot be certain about the year she got a new father. Mohini Varde, Rukhmabai's grand-niece and biographer, records 5 March 1870 as the date of Jayantibai's marriage with Sakharam Arjun. This was two and a half years after the death of her first husband in mid-1867. Considering that Varde provides a precise date, is privy to the family's lore, and has done research for her book, the date would merit serious consideration. However, in a letter dated 17 February 1887, Rukhmabai herself maintained that the marriage took place six years after the death of her biological father, that is, in 1873. She can be implicitly trusted for this date. For, unlike in the case of her date of birth, nothing was to be gained or lost from the year of her mother's remarriage.

Whether Rukhmabai was born in 1863 or 1865 – or 1864, which is not improbable – would today appear inconsequential. So also would the dispute whether she was married at eleven or thirteen. In either case it would remain for us an instance of child marriage. But in Rukhmabai's time the difference between eleven and thirteen was critical. That was a time when the question of the age of consent – the minimum age when a girl could consent to sexual intercourse – was beginning to agitate public opinion. Behramji Malabari, the great crusader for women's cause, had launched his agitation for raising the age of consent. He was demanding that the age be raised from ten to twelve. That is what, in the event that it was enacted, the Age of Consent Act (1891) would provide. Given that twelve was the critical cut-off year in the contemporary debate over child marriage, much seemed to hang for Rukhmabai on showing that she was married at eleven, and for Dadaji on showing that she was thirteen at that time.

Nor is the time when Jayantibai married Sakharam Arjun inconsequential. Whenever it happened, Rukhmabai had to cope with the stress of moving into new surroundings with a stepfather and a step-grandmother. It mattered whether it happened in 1870, when she was five-and-a-half, or in 1873, when she was eight-and-a-half. Rukhmabai – believing the date given by her – was at least lucky that she had to make those difficult adjustments as an eight-and-a-half-year old, not a child three years younger.

2

Quiet Making of a Rebel

RUKHMABAI'S NAME TAKES US REFLEXIVELY to her epochal defiance. That defiance is why we remember her today. It was a defiance that caught everyone off guard. It had to come about for people to believe that it was possible. It may as well have not come about. For years Rukhmabai had vacillated between fear and determination, despair and hope, uncertainty and clarity. She could have chosen either way. A different choice, and the world would not have heard her name.

For years, like the other girls, she was docile and diffident. She did dream of getting educated and carving out a different kind of life; so would have many other girls of the day. She differed in that she made her life radically different. But there was nothing pre-ordained about it. Till very late it seemed that she might end up like the other girls. To recognize this is not to belittle Rukhmabai's resolve which was, without doubt, out of the ordinary. It is, rather, to avoid futile romanticizing. Nothing is easier, and more tempting, than to make Rukhmabai larger than the objective forces around her. But individual successes are never entirely independent of historical constraints.

Rukhmabai grew up in a world that was astir with new ideas. These new ideas were in clash with traditional beliefs and institutions. Reform and orthodoxy were locked in a bitter unending wrangle. It was a very complex, confusing and dynamic world. Orthodoxy and reform, old and new, progressive and reactionary, tradition and change were, of course, words employed to describe that world. They were, no less, also weapons that the rival groups hurled at one another.

As descriptive terms, they concealed as much as they revealed of that world. We have seen in the last chapter that both Sakharam and Ranade were proponents of reform. But, as real flesh-and-blood human beings, neither of them was exclusively new or old, reformer or reactionary. They were both. To further complicate things, there were varying ways in which individuals were both new and old, reformer and reactionary. Ranade was more new with regard to women's education; Sakharam was more new in supporting widow remarriage. We have also seen that Rukhmabai was impacted more by Sakharam's real-life ambivalences than by his categorical progressive precepts.

Similarly, her ideas were also shaped by what she saw of the emerging world of social reform. This was not a distant, impersonal world. She was, for better and worse, located in the thick of it and felt simultaneously enthused and disillusioned about it.

The details of what she studied at home are not known. We have no idea of the books, newspapers and magazines she read. Her readings, probably, were random and miscellaneous, not organized along some kind of a private syllabus. She used to struggle to make sense of her father's books, lectures and newspaper writings. Mohini Varde quotes Rukhmabai as saying: 'I tried to read my father's books and lecture notes but could understand very little.'[1] This struggle was not confined to her father's writings. She would also go through other texts that were above her level of comprehension.

These random readings apart, she and her half-sister, Rani, were often taken along by Sakharam to his public lectures. In addition to providing new information, the lectures and ensuing discussions would instil in Rukhmabai a sense of the culture and significance of public debate. And, of course, she had access to that unique source of learning and reflection: frequent meetings at her place of public men, writers and reformers. She would secretly imagine being like them one day.

Unlike formal schooling, on which Rukhmabai had lost out and which spoon-fed its beneficiaries, her otherwise cumbersome self-education brought her a special advantage. It obliged her to sift and organize the bits and fragments of miscellaneous information, values and ideas that she tirelessly kept accumulating. And this exercise, in turn, helped her forge her own ways of seeing, questioning, arguing and thinking.

Growing up in cheerless isolation was an endless internal polylogue for this inquisitive girl. She was quick to realize that the cheerlessness of her existence was socially ordained. It was the cheerlessness of all her Indian sisters. She was human enough to permit herself the comfort of self-pity and paranoia. But she never permitted herself the delusion that her suffering as a girl-woman was uniquely her own. Every time she provided an account of her life, she framed it within the larger context of the sisterhood. She saw in her own predicament a community of suffering, and in that suffering a larger cause and duty.

Far and near, all around she saw girls inflicted by variations of her own unwarranted and needless suffering. Living next door was her best friend, Shanta. Daughter of the eminent Sanskrit scholar R. G. Bhandarkar, Shanta was eleven when she was married to the son of another prominent public figure of western India, Dr Bhau Daji. Two years later she lost her husband, and came to live with her father. Sorrowing Shanta and Rukhmabai began confiding in each other their intimate thoughts and feelings.

Shanta's case showed Rukhmabai that subtle working of orthodoxy which virtually neutralized the possibility of resistance by its victims. Widow Shanta was fortunate that she was Bhandarkar's daughter and Bhau Daji's daughter-in-law, both stalwart reformers. In 1869, when Bombay's first widow marriage was organized in the wake of the Hindu Widow Remarriage Act of 1855, Bhandarkar was among those who defied organized Hindu orthodoxy and attended the wedding.

Bhau Daji did something remarkable even earlier. In 1862 a public debate was organized to resolve the question of widow marriage. Among the representatives of the reform party in the debate was Karsandas Mulji (1832–71), one of western India's pioneering social reformers. The orthodox party was led by Brijratanji Maharaja, the chief of a Vaishnava sect. The debate, predictably, ended in a deadlock. Thereupon, writing in his *Satya Prakash*, Karsandas charged that the Vaishnava Maharajas had 'wilfully altered to their own advantage the fundamental rules and practices of their religion' and 'systematically perverted their actual position (which in the eyes of their bigoted followers is that of deified humanity) to the most gross and infamous debauchery'.

This provoked Brijratanji to file a libel suit against Karsandas. In his deposition before Justice Joseph Arnould of the Bombay High Court, Karsandas elaborated the charges:

> … all the Maharajas have carnal intercourse with the wives and daughters of their more zealous devotees. Girls are sent to the Maharajas before being touched by their husbands … During the 'Ras' festival, wives and husbands collect promiscuously in a room, and have carnal intercourse promiscusouly among them. The 'Ras' festival is held three or four times in a month. The Maharaja has actual sexual intercourse with many women.

Passions ran high as the Maharaja Libel Case created a sharp split within Hindu society. In that charged atmosphere Dr Bhau Daji proferred a testimony that facilitated the Maharaja's indictment and Karsandas's acquittal. Bhau Daji testified that he had treated Brijratanji Maharaja for syphilitic ulcer on the *glans penis*. Further, that he had, besides Brijratanji, treated two more Maharajas for venereal diseases.

Shanta's mother, Annapoorna Bhandarkar, was no less liberal than her illustrious husband. No Hindu widow could have had such a mother, father and father-in-law. They all pressed her to marry again. In vain. Neither their emotional pleadings nor shastric defence of widow marriage moved Shanta. She was held back by a potent fusion of that amorphous sentiment called *sanskar* – the venerable ideal of a good Hindu wife – and the emotional bond she felt for her deceased boy-husband and for her loving father-in-law, Bhau Daji. Even before making her his daughter-in-law, Bhau Daji had, as her father's friend, showered upon Shanta great warmth and affection. He died suddenly in 1874, and that further deepened her feeling that if she married again she would be betraying her dear departed one.

Bhandarkar and Annapoornabai did not give in. The wise savant worked over the years to bring home to his daughter – like only he could with his mastery of the shastras – the dharmic validity of remarriage. He also invoked Bhau Daji's intrepid commitment to reform to convince Shanta that her remarriage would bring peace to her loving father-in-law's soul. She agreed at last.

Shanta's saga brought young Rukhmabai face to face with a predicament that was diametrically different from her own. She was dreaming dreams that, given the state of Hindu society, were hard to realize. She was let down by an enlightened man. Here was Shanta letting down her enlightened parents who were desperate for her to begin a new life.

This was Rukhmabai's introduction to the baffling complexity of women's predicament. No matter how privileged, a girl was willy-nilly a captive of orthodoxy. All girls – in Rukhmabai's distressing description – were born to be 'enslaved daughters.' How did that happen? Grappling with the question made her understanding of women's predicament acute and nuanced.

She could see from personal experience that the fate of these enslaved daughters depended in a big way on the behaviour of reformers, which was notoriously contradictory. In 1873 she learnt of Ranade betraying the cause of widow remarriage. The following year Vishnu Shastri Pandit (1827–76), founder of the Punarvivahottejak Mandal – Association for Promoting Widow Remarriage – justified his reputation as the Vidyasagar of western India by marrying Kusabai, a widow. Rukhmabai's disappointment of the previous year gave way to elation. She even felt a personal pride, for Vishnu Shastri Pandit was among Sakharam's regular visitors. Unending oscillation between elation and depression became part of Rukhmabai's coming of age. It set her thinking. What lay behind such frustrating uncertainties and behavioural divergences? What could be done to ensure that there was convergence, not divergence, in the profession and practice of reformers? How could victims of social evils be persuaded to respond to progressive influences instead of succumbing to prevailing conventions and expectations?

Her native intelligence and sensitivity sharpened by the unkindness of life, Rukhmabai started writing on the question of women's awakening from her self-study days. In fact, she began doing this even before Behramji Merwanji Malabari, the great crusader for women's emancipation, came out with his celebrated twin 'Notes' on 'Infant Marriage in India' and 'Enforced Widowhood'. Referring to her two pseudonymous letters to the *Times of India*, she claimed:

As regards the sentiments of [those] letters, I had been writing to vernacular papers *on this very subject*, long before Mr Malabari brought them into prominence.[2]

We may not know exactly how 'long before' Malabari did

Rukhmbai begin writing for the Marathi press. But considering that Malabari's 'Notes' were written in August 1884, when Rukhmabai was around twenty, she must have started very young. The silently nursed urge to be like the fine minds she had admired from a distance was clearly at work.

Beginning before Malabari would mean that she began writing around the same time that some other remarkable young women pioneers did. The year 1882 was particularly prolix in this regard. Early in that year appeared Tarabai Shinde's *Stree-Purush Tulana* – 'Comparison of Women and Men' – a text that marks the beginning of a radical feminist critique in India. Later that year, in June, came Pandita Ramabai's *Stree Dharma Neeti*. Just three months later, Ramabai gave her famous testimony before the Hunter Commission, explaining what held Indian women in bondage and suggesting ways for their emancipation. The same year Ramabai Ranade made her debut as a speaker. Unrecognizable from the illiterate ten-year-old nondescript who had entered the Ranade household as the famous man's spouse, this new Ramabai broke free of convention and delivered her maiden public lecture on social reform. And did that in English. 1882 also saw the publication, in faraway Lahore, of *Seemantini Upadesh* by 'Agyaat Hindu Aurat', an uncanny intimation of 'A Hindu Lady', the pseudonym Rukhmabai would assume three years later.

Young, aware women were beginning to realize that they could not leave their cause to the male reformers. Women had to speak up for women.

1882 was also the year Pandita Ramabi founded the Arya Mahila Samaj in Poona. In November of the same year a branch of the Samaj was opened in Bombay and young Rukhmabai chosen as its secretary. Around the same time she also got associated with the Prarthana Samaj. Inspired by the Brahmo Samaj of Bengal, the Prarthana Samaj was a male preserve until it was given a new orientation following the visit to Bombay of Pratap Chandra Mazumdar, a missionary of the Brahmo Samaj. Mazumdar encouraged the leaders of the Prarthana Samaj to formally admit women. Sakharam was prominent among those who backed this reformist innovation. That brought Rukhmabai in close association with the Samaj. Ever eager to learn, she rarely missed the special lectures the Samaj organized for women every Sunday. We have a first-hand description of these meetings by Kashibai Kanitkar. Recalling that Rukhmabai attended the meetings most regularly, Kashibai writes:

> It was more like a class at which one of the Prarthana Samaj members would give a talk on a topic of general interest and provide useful information … The talks covered various social, religious, scientific, and other topics.[3]

Another important exposure that expanded Rukhmabai's horizon and sharpened her thinking came through her acquaintance with some of Bombay's prominent European ladies. Liberal in their outlook, these ladies wanted to contribute their mite to the welfare of Indians, particularly Indian women. One of these, Nora Scott, we have already met in the last chapter. Then there was Dr Edith Pechey at whose place and initiative Nora and Rukhmabai had met.

That was in June 1884. The following year Bombay got an exceptionally liberal governor, Lord Reay. He and his wife were particularly interested in the cause of women. For her part, Lady Reay started organizing zenana parties by way of promoting enlightenment and better interracial relations. To these parties were invited European ladies and ladies belonging to different Indian communities. Sakharam's social position secured young Rukhmabai an entry to those parties and her personality made sure that she was invited regularly.

Apart from expanding her mental horizon and allaying her

natural diffidence, Lady Reay's parties gave Rukhmabai a chance to converse in English. Here is an interesting anecdote Rukhmabai herself reported:

I used to be invited to the ladies' parties of the Government house. At that time, my knowledge of English was inadequate. For example, when Mrs Solomon Sassoon came to talk to me, I said to her, 'Are you Mrs S. Sassoon? I did not know you were the same thing.' As a practical joke, she took me to Lady Reay and told her that I called her a 'thing.'[4]

Edith Pechey deserves the most special mention in this biography. The many ways in which she helped Rukhmabai will unfold by and by in this narrative. Meanwhile, we may hear Rukhmabai herself about her exemplar and benefactor:

... when my trials began in 1884, Dr. Pechey took up my cause in real earnest, and worked very hard in interesting other people to form a committee in my defense ... She was my mainstay for sympathy and support all through the long weary four years of my trials, and she constantly urged me to proceed to England and study Medicine ... It did not take long to convert me to her views, but the difficulty lay with my mother and grandfather. Even now it is not an easy matter for a Hindu to cross the 'black waters' ... twenty years ago it was almost impossible. But all these difficulties were overcome by her tact and perseverance ... When I finished my studies and qualified, in 1894, it was Dr. Pechey-Phipson who secured a position of Medical Officer for me at Surat, and my little quarters there are full of mementoes of her kind thought of me. Last year [1907] when I wrote to her about a Lecture scheme for the women of Surat, she at once took up the idea, and though ill herself, she spared no trouble in writing to friends and collecting funds for my object ... She was the great champion of women, and hundreds of grateful women in India can testify to her kind acts for their welfare.[5]

What was it about this woman that made her a role model for Rukhmabai? Thirty-eight-year-old Dr Pechey landed in Bombay on 12 December 1883 to be at the helm of the newly launched Medical Women for India movement. She was one of the seven women who, hard on the heels of Elizabeth Garrett Anderson, the first woman to obtain a British licence to practise medicine, had mounted the first organized offensive against men's monopoly over the medical profession.

The offensive was orchestrated by a fiery young woman named Sophia Jex-Blake. She applied for admission to the medical course at the London University and was, expectedly, denied admission. Then she applied at the University of Edinburgh to be told that it was not advisable for the university to make alterations 'in the interest of one lady'. Sophia thereupon issued a public call, asking other women to join her in seeking medical education. Edith Pechey was the first to respond, and she was joined in by three others: Isabel Thorne, Matilda Chaplin, Helen Evans. Celebrated as the 'Edinburgh Five', they were soon joined in by Mary Anderson and Emily Bovell, for the group to be rechristened the 'Edinburgh Seven'.

All seven women did exceedingly well in the preliminary examination. Out of 152 candidates, four women were among the top seven. From then on, the women's performance was outstanding at every stage. Yet – in fact, for that reason – throughout they were constantly harassed and hampered by many of their anti-women teachers and fellow students, as evidenced in this account of an incident, aptly called the 'Edinburgh Riot', by Dr Louisa Martindale:

As the five women walked down to the Surgeons' Hall to their examination, a dense mob greeted them. Not a single policeman was in sight and the crowd was sufficient to stop the traffic for an hour. When they arrived at the gates, a number of young medical students, fortified by whisky and using foul language, shut the gates in their faces. The women students waited quietly on the steps until suddenly one of their fellow students rushed forward and wrenched open the gates in spite of the howls of the half-tipsy students, and they were able to pass through and sit through their examination ... At the end of the examination, a lecturer offered to let them out by the back door. They refused and immediately twenty or thirty students, most of them Irish, formed a bodyguard so that the little procession passed through the howling crowd, and, except for mud and rotten eggs and torn dresses, reached their homes to safety. This, of course, was not the end and a few weeks later there came the publication of a host of indecent articles in various papers.[6]

Those brave female pioneers were variously harassed inside the class rooms, in the university and also outside in the city. They were pitted against the petty cunning of men ensconced in positions of power and determined to repel the women's invasion. Edith Pechey, for instance, scored the highest marks in chemistry at the end of the first year's examination and was entitled to a prize – the Hope Prize – of two thousand pound sterling and free access to the chemistry laboratory (at a time when women students were denied entry to the laboratory). Edith was denied the prize which was, instead, given to a male student who was second in the order of merit.

The university authorities tried to cover up this gender-induced injustice, arguing that Edith Pechey was not entitled to the prize because the women students were not members of the regular class; they had studied at a different hour. The authorities later gave away their own little game twice over by letting Edith Pechey have the bronze medal to which her marks had entitled her, and all the women students their certificates of attendance.

Ironically, all that harassment, persecution and discrimination was touted as being for women's good. 'Admitting women in the ranks of medicine,' it was claimed, 'is derogatory to the status and character of the female sex.'

To cut a fascinating story short, just when the brave battlers were about to succeed after five years of determined struggle, the university expelled them in 1874 on the ground that it – the university – had 'exceeded its authority' by granting them admission in the first instance. As a last recourse, the women approached the High Court of Scotland. The court's final verdict, by a single vote, was against them. The court even ordered them to pay the university the legal costs. They were saved from ruin by the enlightened among Edinburgh's citizens. Incensed by the female students' persecution, the citizens had formed a Committee to Secure a Complete Medical Education for Women in Edinburgh soon after the denial of the Hope Prize to Edith Pechey. The committee issued a public appeal for financial and moral support, and the university was paid its costs.

Three years after their expulsion, Edith Pechey and Sophia Jex-Blake obtained their M.D. from the University of Berne in 1877.

But going out to obtain a degree was no answer to the question of medical education for women in Britain. The ever-intrepid Sophia Jex-Blake now set about establishing an independent institution to train women in medicine. This brought into being, in 1874, the London School of Medicine for Women. That is where Rukhmabai would later go for her medical education. Also, she would get her first medical degree – Triple Qualification – from the same University of Edinburgh that had expelled its first female medical students, and stay with the legendary Sophia Jex-Blake in Edinburgh.

The saga of the Edinburgh Seven made a deep impact on Rukhmabai. While still reading Sophia Jex-Blake's stirring account of the saga, *Medical Women: Two Essays*, which Pechey had lent her, Rukhmabai confided to Pechey:

It is so very interesting to me that I don't like to drop a single word of it while reading. It gives me a great comfort as I see the truth won the victory at last, though you had to suffer so much even in a country like Europe [sic]. I would never have believed if some common person were to tell me, that the people there were so against to allow women to study medicine ...

This was in June 1886, when Rukhmabai herself was being harassed and hounded. She was in that hour of trial buoyed up by Jex-Blake's blow-by-blow account of the trial the 'Edinburgh Seven' went through, and by having one of the seven, Pechey, by her side. She would recall years later:

> ... when my trials began in 1884, Dr Pechey took up my cause in real earnest, and worked very hard in interesting other people to form a committee in my defence ... She was my mainstay for sympathy and support all through the four years of my trial ...[7]

Pechey did much more, and well beyond those four years. Identifying instinctively with Rukhmabai, Pechey felt compelled to stand up with the young crusader. She also realized that the girl, for all her fire and determination, needed not only unstinted support during her trial but also gentle counselling to help her overcome her educational deficiencies and have a secure independent future. Pechey knew she had to be the girl's guardian angel.

Consider, for example, the thought that prompted Pechey to loan such utterly different books as *A Roman Singer* and *Medical Women* to Rukhmabai at the height of the controversy that raged around her case. The loan of *A Roman Singer*, a popular novel about an Italian tenor's love for the daughter of a Prussian officer, was obviously meant to counter the prospect of young Rukhmabai becoming, to borrow her own expression, cold to 'love matters'. Pechey's move, as we have seen in the previous chapter, did not have the desired result. But the fact that she made the thoughtful gesture shows that she cared for Rukhmabai, the person, not merely for a cause.

We have no idea of what Rukhmabai thought and said at the time she started writing for the Marathi press. To understand her mind, we have to rely on the little that she wrote in English. Her first piece was a long letter in the *Times of India* of 26 June 1885. Appearing under a pseudonym, 'A Hindu Lady', the letter was a veritable essay on the intertwined problems of infant/child marriage and enforced widowhood within the larger context of the depressing state of women in India. Rukhmabai began with a disarming confession, saying:

Not being accustomed to writing in English – particularly to newspapers – I submitted this letter to the inspection of a friend who has kindly looked over and corrected it, where he thought corrections were necessary ... I have to thank this gentleman not only for the literary help given by him, but also for the genuine sympathy he feels for our condition.

There is no docility or diffidence in the confession. It has, rather, the honesty and humility of one who knows she has something important to say. In fact, honesty and humility would all her life remain essential characteristics of her magnetic personality. There is also in the confession a happy readiness to express gratitude where gratitude is due. Thus, referring to her theme – infant marriage and enforced widowhood – Rukhmabai acknowledges in the very second paragraph of the letter:

The above subjects have been very keenly discussed throughout India for the last few months. The agitation against these evil customs is mainly due to the exertions of Mr Malabari, who has laid all Indian women under a debt of gratitude, for which we cannot thank him too much.

Gratitude expressed, Rukhmabai commences her analysis with an emphatic statement about the gravity of the problem. She says:

Everybody knows the misery, which is brought upon the Hindu Community by these wicked institutions. Misery which is not confined to any particular class or section but affects all alike – the rich and the poor, the old and young.

The misery, she stresses, is not confined to women. It also impacts men, even though 'it tells most heavily upon the female sex'. It affects 'the whole community'.

She is baffled that even as foreigners are moved by this misery, 'why do our own people shut their eyes and remain as indifferent and unconcerned as ever?' Her question is rhetorical, a preface for the following indictment:

The cause of this apathy seems to me to be this – that either our people have no real desire to introduce wholesome reforms in our social customs or they have no moral courage to endure the difficulties in which such reforms may temporarily land them.

Rukhmabai explicates the charge in the rest of the letter. Hers is no ordinary explication. It is an explication by one who has personally suffered that which she is explicating. She speaks as a witness who feels justified in delivering her verdict also.

To begin with, she shows that the misery caused by evil social customs tells most heavily on the female sex:

Hindu social customs do not entail upon men half of the difficulties which they entail upon women ... Marriage does not interpose any insuperable obstacle in the course of their studies. They can marry, not only a second wife on the death of the first, but have the right of marrying any number of wives at the same time, if they please. If married early, they are not called upon to go to the house and submit to the tender mercies of a mother-in-law. Nor is any restraint put upon their action because of their marriage. But in case of women, it is the very opposite of this ...

Pointing out that most girls are married around the age of eight and, as an inevitable sequel, deprived of education, Rukhmabai continues:

Thus, Mr Editor, when we are just beginning to appreciate education, we are taken away from school and, therefore, you can imagine what progress, if any, we could make in our studies in the scanty time at our disposal ...

There are, she says, some reformers around, but their number 'is insignificantly small'. Besides, even if a handful of them 'dared to oppose the prejudices of their community' and continued the schooling of their daughters and daughters-in-law after marriage, that hardly helped the child-wife:

For, she is generally a mother before she is fourteen, when she must, of sheer necessity, give up the dream of mental cultivation and face hard realities of life. It seems, therefore, hopeless to expect any advancement in the higher female education, when the custom of infant, or rather, early marriage continues as rife as before. Unless the state of things changes, all the efforts at higher female education seems like putting the cart before the horse.

Not only early motherhood and denial of education, nearly everything about life in the husband's family, which perforce became the married woman's home, guaranteed 'loss of mental and physical freedom'. Rukhmabai backs her description of the poor wife's predicament with a wealth of disturbing details, and, in doing that, breaks, uncharacteristically, into angry sarcasm:

She must never think of sitting or speaking in the presence of her father-in-law or mother-in-law, nay, even in the presence of any other member of their family. She must get up early and go to bed late. Must work with the servants. (I do not say like the servants, for they have the option of refusing to work, which she has not.) It is the undoubted privilege of the mother-in-law to find fault with everything and anything done by the unfortunate victim. Any remonstrance from the culprit is promptly and sharply met by a torrent of abuse, often followed by direct or indirect corporal chastisement. If this discipline does not make the girl as docile as a beast, and as submissive as a slave, the mother-in-law can use her last weapon and turn the girl out of door. This is an extreme to which the girl, if she is wise, will not drive her mother-in-law to resort. For she can find no sympathy or protection in her distress from her parents, who might be regarded as the natural guardians, if she is ignominiously turned out. They angrily advise her to forthwith repair to her husband's house and make due amends to the all-powerful mother-in-law. No help need be expected from the husband … Even if he has the will he has not the power to help his wife out of the misery.

Having brought into public view the miserable existence into which women were thrown early in their lives, Rukhmabai hammers home the conclusion that this is designed to make the poor woman 'timid, languid, melancholy, sickly, devoid of cheerfulness, and therefore incapable of communicating to others'.

Further, insofar as customs derived their sanction from religion, Rukhmabai savages the ancient law-givers. The shastra-givers, she insists, were male and just did not have it in them to be even-handed and equitable. They believed themselves – as men – to be pure and blameless, and 'laid every conceivable sin and impurity at our door'.

Our door! This – women's door – is central to Rukhmabai's understanding. She recognizes a fundamental divide between 'us' – 'the female sex' – and 'them', 'our' blindly self-righteous male exploiters. That is why not only the law-givers but men in general 'cannot, in the least, understand the wretchedness which we Hindu women have to endure':

> If these worthies are to be trusted, we are a set of unclean animals created by God for the special service and gratification of man, who by right divine can treat or maltreat us at his own sweet will. Reduced to this state of degradation by the dictum of the Shastras, looked down upon for ages by men, we have naturally come to look down upon ourselves.

Rukhmabai wanted that men also must see the bane of gender divide.

It is noteworthy that Rukhmabai squarely faces the tragic reality of women's mindless participation in their own degradation. But it is radically different from men's self-serving blasé representation of the same phenomenon. Recall, for confirmation, her own father's specious justification for the yawning divide between their practice and profession:

> How many of our vaunted reformers have had to eat their own words to meekly practise in private what they eloquently denounced in public because their wives and mothers, sisters and cousins proved too strong for them.

No less significantly, Rukhmabai exposes the myth that 'the advent of the English' had initiated 'a great activity in the direction of reform'. Whatever might be the fruits of that activity, 'there is not the least general improvement in social or domestic life of the natives, at least of the Hindus'. Without women, too, benefiting from that civilizing process, there can only be educated individuals, not families that are 'educated as a whole'. Men educated in English, Rukhmabai argues, cannot be expected to, in turn, educate women in their own families. The most enlightened of them, even those who cried hoarse about women's education, had little to show by way of actual action. Showing how the horse and the cart ought to be positioned, she writes:

Our condition, therefore, cannot, Sir, be improved unless the practice of early marriages is abolished, and higher female education is largely disseminated.

The preliminary imperative step, she asserts, is to legislate away the 'wicked custom':

I have been thinking, Sir, for a long time, of some means by which we could escape the grinding thraldom of this wicked custom. And the only efficient remedy that suggested itself to me was to appeal to the Government to come to our help and to root out this pernicious custom which is eating up the very core of Hindu society.

At this point in her letter, she brings in Malabari yet again. She had for long thought that governmental action alone could better the lot of women. But she had kept silent because there was little chance 'for a poor helpless woman like me to successfully approach and get redress from an august body like the Government'. She was 'almost giving way to despair' when Malabari came out with his 'Notes', and the Government promptly responded by inviting 'the opinions of the leaders of the Hindu society'. Her despair was gone, for a while at any rate:

> I felt sure that now these gentlemen were aroused to the sense of their duty, they would join in a body and strengthen the hands of Government in ameliorating the condition of their daughters and sisters. But, alas! For the pleasing delusion! The opinions of most of these gentlemen, which have been permitted to see the light, have dashed my hope to pieces.

Rukhmabai fears that the government would be wary of legislating in the face of opposition from those whom it viewed as the leaders of Hindu society. But this time, instead of lapsing back into despair and silence, she exposes the hollowness of the arguments advanced against Malabari. Having already exposed those who spoke the language of reform and pretended to be women's well-wishers – 'so called men of light & learning' – she first lists their objections to Malabari's 'Notes': that Malabari, not being Hindu, has no business to meddle with the affairs of Hindus; that abolition of infant marriage would promote 'vice'; 'that gradual spread of education would bring about the necessary changes in fifty or sixty years'; that infant/early marriage is not harmful 'provided consummation is put off for a sufficiently long period'; and that seeking government help in social matters is 'a humiliation', and 'in courting legislative interference we shall be endangering our freedom of action'.

Rukhmabai dismisses these objections as 'a trifle too specious', and insists that 'unless the Government puts a stop to the custom of early marriage, our people are not likely, for centuries together, to abolish it'. She queries caustically:

Do these gentlemen think that the Government was not right in abolishing Sati and infanticide fifty years ago? And that it should have waited till we were sufficiently enlightened to see the iniquities and had abolished them ourselves?

And continues with unsparing sarcasm:

It is, Sir, all very well to talk loudly of education and enlightenment and so on till no sacrifice or duty is required from those who boast of them. Can any of these gentlemen honestly tell us what enlightenment they have introduced, or even tried to introduce? If, Sir, educated men like these, who fully admit the existence of the evils, have neither the pluck nor the strong sense of duty to fight them, need we wonder at the indifference of the uneducated masses? In a society where the educated, or the 'upper ten' are indifferent and the uneducated ignorant, is it rash to invoke Government aid for the redress of these crying grievances?

However, Rukhmabai is unhappy with Malabari's extreme caution in proposing legislative interference. Rather than propose a minimum age for marriage, he had merely proposed an increase in the age of consent; that, too, from the existing ten to twelve years. Persuaded that this paltry change would achieve nothing, Rukhmabai suggests the following measures:

1. Any marriage performed without the sanction of Government, if disputed within a certain period, shall be null and void.
2. That no marriage shall be legal unless the bride is 15 and the bridegroom is 20 years old.
3. After the passing of this law, if any man be married before 20, he shall forfeit his right to enter the university. (This provision

need not be rigorously enforced for some time as it may punish children for the sins of their parents).

4. Just as in large towns and cities registers of births and deaths, and in Bombay registers of vaccination, are kept, and any neglect is punished by fine, there shall be registers kept for marriages. And if the married are under the age sanctioned by law, they or their parents shall be liable for punishment.

5. If it is found that parents have laid a tax on, or in other words sold their daughters, they shall be punished by law.

She proposes a sixth measure also, which we have discussed in the first chapter in the context of Rukhmabai's harrowing encounter with Narayan Dhurmaji: 'Under no circumstances shall the wife be older than the husband.'

Finally, despite her deep distrust of them, Rukhmabai entreats 'the leaders of our community to consider the matter in solemn and fair spirit'. Hoping against hope, to shame them and sting their conscience, she addresses them directly:

If we do not complain of misery entailed upon us by the evil custom of early marriage, it does not follow that our misery is less acute than it really is. If a poverty stricken man puts up with many privations and inconveniences which could not be borne by people who are very well off, it does not follow that the former does not suffer, only because he does not complain. I pray, therefore, do not think that our misery is light because we are inured to it. Because you cannot see our hurt feelings, do not think that we have no taste or aspiration for a better life.

You gentlemen anxiously long for the regeneration of India. If arts and science flourish, and if trade and industry progress among our people, you think everything will be right. India will prosper. But do you seriously believe (I beseech you to consider calmly) that such a happy state of things is possible when you allow boys and girls to be fathers and mothers before they are hardly out of their teens? Do you expect anything good or great from a young boy or girl saddled with the cares and anxieties of an increasing family, and having to fight their way through the hard realities of life?

Angry though she felt about the cavernous divide between men and women, Rukhmabai had the sense to realize that the well-being of both required harmony between them. If, therefore, she needed to reach out to men, her stance had to be non-antagonistic. She had to speak of both the sons and the daughters, of men as well as women. Also, despite her wholesale castigation of the male law-givers of yore, she had to make use of the belief in India's glorious past. All this comes together in her stirring concluding appeal:

> I entreat you, gentlemen, once more, before this newly awakened desire for social reform wanes, to co-operate with the Government in emancipating your sons and daughters from the social thraldom under which they grow. If you succeed in bringing about this salutary reform of education, development of arts and science, the production of an able bodied and strong minded race of men and women – in fact the mental and material prosperity of India – will follow as a matter of course, and India will revert to its once proud position in the scale of nations.

Rukhmabai had in this letter set out to discuss the twin problems of infant/early marriage and enforced widowhood. But the discussion of early marriage alone had become so long that she had to end it abruptly. Moreover, she had meant, after her appeal to the leaders of society, to conclude with an 'appeal on behalf of myself and my suffering sisters, to His Excellency, the Viceroy, to devote a portion of his precious time to the consideration of this subject'. That, too, she could not do for reasons of space.

To the pending question of enforced widowhood Rukhmabai returned three months later. Mocking the shastras for being 'eminently equitable' in treating 'the young and the old alike', she began by laying bare the enormity of the evil of enforced widowhood. According to the shastras, she wrote:

> ... if a girl, I should say a child of five or six, married for the gratification of her parents, who hardly knows the meaning of the words 'husband and wife', 'wifedom' or 'widowhood', has been so unfortunate as to lose her child-husband, [she] is, according to the incorrigible Hindu law, as much a widow as a grandmother who loses her man at the ripe old age of 70!

Then she turned from the shastras to pour her boiling scorn on her contemporaries:

> I commend the even-handed justice of our religious rulers to those who can appreciate it. But as far as I am concerned, it shocks my feelings by its vivid contrast and obvious iniquity. I wonder, reputed as Hindus are, and I think justly, for their mild humanity, what perverse blindness warped the judgment of these earlier writers that made them lose sight of the great difference between the condition of a child-widow of six and a matron-widow of sixty? How brutalised must have been human nature when it could stamp an innocent mite with the dreadful epithet 'widow' and provide for her that lifelong misery which is the inevitable lot of Hindu widows?

Showing – 'There is no use in mincing matters' – what men's brutalization could make them do to their women, Rukhmabai continues:

> ... these locks, the pride of young women, are ruthlessly sheared at the instigation of the butcher-priest ... Her presence is shunned.

She is a leper of society, doomed to pass her life in seclusion and not allowed to mix freely with her people. If the unfortunate creature unwittingly intrudes her odious presence on any occasion of joy or festivity, the company curses her presence and regards it as an evil omen, sure to be followed by some great calamity ... [T]his company is mostly composed of her dear and near relatives.

She must put on coarse garments and eat unsavoury food and that too, as happens in many families, only once a day. The menial work of the family becomes her lot as a matter of course. She must observe all the fasts of which the Hindu calendar is very prolific.

Having tried anger and sarcasm, Rukhmabai lectures her countrymen:

I entreat my countrymen to be judge of the miseries of widows by transferring the same penalties to men. Suppose, it has been enacted that when a man lost his wife he should continue celibate, live on coarse fare, be tabooed from society, should continue to wear mourning beads for the remainder of his life and practise whether he would or not, never-ending austerities ... [W]ould my countrymen not have long since revolted against such inhuman treatment? ... [I]s it decent, is it human, to make poor helpless ignorant women the victims of a system, the like of which has not disgraced any civilised society?

The reference here to women's ignorance is a reminder of its connection with the custom of early marriage and enforced widowhood. In just one sentence Rukhmabai sums up what the widow's ignorance does:

Her ignorance makes her entirely depend upon the pittance, which her male relatives would be pleased to dole out to her, and she must drag on her existence, as best as she can, in agony of mind and body.

Rukhmabai knows that her countrymen are inured to the pervasive iniquity and injustice of their laws. Left to themselves, they would not recognize the egregious wrongs done to women through the 'gentle decrees' of their 'human legislators'. She must show them what they have done. Instances, she chides her countrymen:

> are not rare of the edifying spectacle of dying, old men, who have had the great misfortune of losing their second or third wife, preparing to play the young bridegroom and sending their men to hunt out a young girl (of ten or eleven) [read *akshat yoni*] to bless the remaining days of their life. And this too, they are in such a hurry to do that the future partner is usually fixed upon ... even before the thirteen conventional days of mourning are over.

Further:

> Now, this same [dying, old] worthy gentleman, who is so solicitous to gratify his vanity (to term it in the mildest way) is philosophically rigid in case of his widowed daughter or grand-daughter, who is just 15 and entering the most critical period of life (when girlhood ends and womanhood begins). The comfort he brings to his sorrowing daughter is in this way. 'My darling,' says the affectionate father, 'fate has ordained this widowhood for you and what human effect can upset the decree of fate! This is the punishment for the sins of your previous birth and you can escape your sins only by leading a life of austerity and devotion. Give up, dear, the vanities of this world and lead a life of purity.' In fact, he exhorts her to be in the world, but not of the world.

'What a charming contrast between noble words and ignoble actions,' expostulates Rukhmabai and warns that 'the laws of nature and society exercise the same influence on man and woman'. She mentions 'a renowned champion of Hinduism, one of our foremost leaders, one who is credited with as much wisdom as learning', who:

> held forth for the noble and pure life which widows of India led, and which, if my memory serves me right, in his opinion was such a balm to their soul, such an incentive to self-abnegation that widowhood was more a blessing than a misfortune from a spiritual point of view! The woes and wails of widows seemed to have no opening to his heart.

So incensed is Rukhmabai by 'this strange native insensibility to the miseries of widows' that she is driven to say: 'I wish (my God, forgive the wish) that he [the champion of Hinduism] had a widowed daughter, or the prospect of having one.'

The storm raging inside her was not just her own. She was speaking for all her voiceless sisters: 'Had the millions of my sisters who are groaning under the miseries of "Perpetual Widowhood" been able to appeal to you and your readers, I should have been only too glad to remain silent.'

Rukhmabai had in her first letter observed that, even if much less in comparison to women, men also were victims of the iniquitous traditional system. She now turned to the question and asked what, besides their selfishness, it was that made Hindu men cling to that system. Her explanation was:

> Custom, I have read somewhere, is the 'Magistrate of a man's life.' If this is a general rule, I should say that custom is a 'full power' magistrate of a Hindu's life. It blinds his judgement, saps the cource of his affections and makes him – though naturally one of the kindliest of human beings – dead to the woes of his daughters and sisters.

The explanation strengthened Rukhmabai's conviction that nothing would happen without legislation:

> To conclude, Sir, the Hindu widow – unbeloved of God and despised of man – a social pariah and domestic drudge, must continue for centuries together to bear her hard portion and pine in solitude till the pressure of legislation or the influence of foreign civilisation comes to her help ...

The letters of 'A Hindu Lady' represent young Rukhmabai at her irreverant and rebellious best. They reflect a maturity of reflection, brilliance of reasoning, and power of articulation far beyond her years. And, of course, courage and freedom from fear. But what makes her voice unique is the ring of truth and suffering. She, as the *Times of India* remarked:

> writes out of the fulness and bitterness of her heart. Countless generations of silent sufferers have found an eloquent exponent at last; and it is impossible to read her letter[s] without being struck with the really lofty tone of her invective, with the virility of her arguments, and, above all, with the indignant scorn she showers upon those who hold that Hindu women have no reason for complaint.[8]

The letters created a great stir. The reaction of the orthodox was violent and abusive. Stung by a 'A Hindu Lady' – a woman speaking for women – they countered that the letters were ghostwritten by a man out to discredit Hindus. In marked contrast, despite their sharp criticism by Rukhmabai, the reformers appreciated her powerful intervention and further broadcast her letters.

In fact, the reformers' sympathetic engagement with the letters of 'A Hindu Lady' led to a significant change in Rukhmabai's position on the question of reform. She had, in the letters, described all ancient law-givers as misogynists and rejected wholesale the laws made by them. Some of the leading lights of social reform, while being fulsome in their praise for 'A Hindu Lady', advised her to study the matter with greater care. Prominent among them was Dewan Bahadur Raghunath Rao (1831–1912). Not knowing that they were the same person, Raghunath Rao lent full support to 'A Hindu Lady' in her impassioned plea for reform and to Rukhmabai in her refusal to go to her husband. But he also advised 'A Hindu Lady' 'to find out whether our Rishis were really as cruel as they have been made to appear'. If she did, he assured her, she would discover that:

> they fully sympathised with you and shared all your views. They say that the family in which the softer sex is not happy brings ruin upon itself. This saying has been fulfilled.[9]

Similarly, *Indu Prakash*, the foremost reformist Anglo-Marathi weekly of Maharashtra, saw where the 'vituperation and sarcastic abuse' of 'A Hindu Lady' vis-à-vis 'the poor old Rishis' came from. It was in their name that the existing oppressive system was justified. But they were, the weekly wrote, 'no more to blame for the hard lot of the modern Hindu widow than the poor widow herself'.[10]

A fast learner, Rukhmabai recognized the validity of the reformers' friendly criticism, and accordingly revised her broad-brush position. Writing less than two years later, she observed:

> Now for the Sastras and the Hindu laws. It is clearly stated in our religious books that a boy … should study for 12 years, and then after having a good experience in the world for four years more

should be allowed to marry at the age of 22 with a girl of suitable age and with his own accord. Well, for girls also it is stated that they should be allowed to marry when they become of age and with their own choice, though nothing has been said for their education. We find in ancient history marriages taking place between the boys and girls of mature age and with their own liking. But these good laws have ceased to be observed and other pernicious customs have taken their place, the results of which lie before us in many horrible forms.[11]

Rukhmabai maintained the same position when, another three years later, she contributed an article, entitled 'Indian Child Marriages: An Appeal to the British Government', to the newly launched London monthly, the *New Review*.[12]

But that did not alter her view of the cruel social system to which women were condemned.

There were many – including some sympathizers – who found the protest of 'A Hindu Lady' marred by exaggeration. Malabari saw the insensitivity of the criticism. In a public rebuke – still relevant for listening to the nascent voices of the disprivileged and the deprived – he lashed out:

It is a sin to talk of exaggeration in the case of a woman who has become frenzied by the cruel injustice which has blighted her life. Here is a language of exaggeration only so far as it is the language of acute suffering ... 'A Hindu Lady' does not belong to that class of reformers who plume themselves upon their scientific accuracy and exactitude, entering upon the decimal fractions of social diseases, with a philosophic calm which can never lead to action ... It is these virtuous, these moderate reformers who are the greatest obstruction in the path of progress. They are so plausible that the stranger is sure to be taken in by their air of impartiality. But it is to this warmth of expression (exaggeration, if you like) and not the trick of concealing one half and explaining away the other half that we owe all important reforms.[13]

'A Hindu Lady', as we shall soon see, was ready to live out her protest to the bitter end.

3

To the High Court

DADAJI'S MOTHER DIED WITHIN FOUR months of his marriage. With that came to grief the plan to make him a good man. Like water finding its level, the nineteen-year-old wastrel spurned the good father-in-law's tutelage and went to live with Narayan Dhurmaji, his maternal uncle and the villain in this story. Two months after this – three months, according to Dadaji – Rukhmabai reached the customary age for *garbhadhan*, the rite that heralds consummation of marriage, which Dr Sakharam stalled on grounds of health.

Initially denied for medical reasons, cohabitation with Rukhmabai continued to elude Dadaji year after year. During those years of separate living, Rukhmabai and Dadaji developed in diametrically opposite directions. That made unbridgeable the divide of class and social background that had existed between them even before the brutal embrace of marriage.

Rukhmabai grew into a cultured, serious-minded and prepossessing young lady. This is how she – Miss Sakharam – is described in Nora Scott's *Journal*:

I was struck by the first sight of her as she sat in her graceful sari talking to Miss Pechey; her whole air was so modest and dignified.

She is 19 years old but looks older, dark brown with a sweet thoughtful face.[1]

The *Times of India* described her as a 'high-spirited woman of refinement, culture and intellectual superiority' who was 'well versed in Western as well as Eastern literature'.[2]

Dadaji, in the meanwhile, deteriorated beyond repair. Such, in fact, was the contrast that Justice Pinhey shuddered at the thought of having to force this woman 'of cultivated taste and possessed of many intellectual gifts and acquirements' into the arms of that 'ignorant journeyman carpenter'. Soon thereafter Latham, one of Rukhmabai's three lawyers, described Dadaji as a 'coolie' in the court of the same Chief Justice Sargent who, as we have seen, could not understand how Rukhmabai was wedded to Dadaji.

This marriage appears foredoomed in hindsight. It did not seem so to the concerned families. Leaving aside the other party's keenness for the match, even Rukhmabai and her people took long to give up on the marriage. They may have sensed trouble when, following his mother's death, Dadaji went to live with Narayan Dhurmaji. But they did not give up. When Dadaji 'was attacked with consumption' and 'not expected to live another season', Sakharam treated him back to life. He even helped Dadaji and his brothers with money for a while. Overlooking Dadaji's persistent rebelliousness, Sakharam kept trying to salvage the marriage. But even he, ultimately, saw the writing on the wall. As Rukhmabai tells us, 'my father, considering his [Dadaji's] constitution, habits, and unfitnes for any work, resolved not to send me to his house to live as his wife'.[3]

Rukhmabai herself took time to write off Dadaji. Though she claimed that she had all along felt 'a great disgust' – indeed, 'natural distaste' – for married life, she, too, for a while hoped for things to improve. She would keep her ears trained for whatever bits of information she could obtain about the man; information regarding his character, the company he kept, his finances, his health, the goings-on in the Narayan Dhurmaji household. She might occasionally get bits that seemed encouraging, but the overall prospect remained depressing. Finally, she also decided, as she put it, to 'wash my hands' of the man.

But Jayantibai and Harishchandra Yadavji were insistent that she should commence a normal marital life. They had no illusions about Dadaji, but they did not want their family honour to be reduced to tatters by their girl's refusal to respect the sacred bond of marriage. Having got an undesirable husband, to their thinking, was no reason to sever the bond. There was, after all, nothing extraordinary about the situation.

Even after the case had been filed in the Bombay High Court, Jayantibai and Harishchandra Yadavji kept pestering Sakharam till his last days to prevail upon Rukhmabai to go and live with Dadaji. For all their pains, they were publicly accused by Dadaji of coveting Rukhmabai's property and not letting her live with him.

Sakharam was indeed responsible for a good deal of Rukhmabai's suffering, and also tended to pass off the responsibility onto the women of the family. But, with Dadaji's incorrigibility surfacing inexorably, Sakharam could no more evade the realization that it was he who had, knowingly or unknowingly, brought Rukhmabai to the brink of ruin. He must, therefore, try and save her. Which he did. And shone at his brightest as a human being, as a father, as a social reformer.

For a while all the three guardians of Rukhmabai were anxious to make her marriage succeed. Even then Sakharam was the one whose anxiety to get the marriage working was tempered the most by concern for Rukhmabai's welfare and feelings in the matter. In fact, even while committing the original sin – but for which there would have been no litigation – he had devised his pre-emptive *ghar jamaai* plan. The same concern also informed the efforts he made under pressure from Jayantibai and Harishchandra Yadavji to effect a compromise and salvage the marriage. And his stalling of Rukhmabai's *garbhadhan* ceremony. This is Dadaji's version of what happened:

> The marriage was not at once consummated because Dr Sakharam Arjun volunteered the opinion that an early consummation would result in the issue of a weak progeny, and he told me this in a friendly way, while I accepted his advice in the same friendly spirit. My wife, Rakhmabai, was therefore, in deference to Dr Sakharam's wish, permitted to remain with her mother and stepfather.[4]

Dadaji, at nineteen, was old enough to consummate the marriage. Sakharam's intervention was clearly for Rukhmabai. He also knew that this would have to be an indefinite postponement. Rukhmabai was not to go to Narayan Dhurmaji's questionable surroundings, and Dadaji was in no mood to be a *ghar jamaai*. It was best to gain time until the couple could live on their own. Or, hoping against hope, Dadaji could be persuaded to change his mind.

For much of the eight years that cohabitation was deferred on one pretext or another, it was a cat-and-mouse game between the rival sides, one pressing for cohabitation, and the other evading it. For a while things unfolded gradually. It was comparatively easy to seek postponement on medical grounds. Dadaji's prolonged illness, and his treatment by Sakharam, left the other side with no option but to bide its time. Then came a point when it ran out of patience.

Sakharam had to walk a tightrope. He saw Dadaji's intransigence and Narayan Dhurmaji's perfidy grow. But he had to keep them in good humour, given the pressure for a compromise – surrender – from Jayantibai and Harishchandra Yadavji. Even after he had decided to go the whole hog with Rukhmabai, there were limits to what he, a stepfather, could do. He had to act diplomatically and quietly neutralize the efforts of Jayantibai and Harishchandra to make the marriage work.

Then the inevitable happened. Their fate was becoming clear to Dadaji and Narayan Dhurmaji. Unless they did something drastic, Rukhmabai's side would keep playing the procrastination game. In any case, already an adult at the time of his marriage, Dadaji was approaching thirty. He had pined long enough to possess his attractive wife and her property. Besides, debts had piled up and, sensing that Rukhmabai might never come to him, the lenders were pressing for repayment and reluctant to loan any more. No less desperate for the couple's cohabitation was Narayan Dhurmaji, the lustful uncle-in-law and debtor-in-chief.

There were also the usual busybodies who had their different reasons to add fuel to the fire. Besides the ones who would not forego the perverse pleasure of a salacious scandal, there were the self-appointed sentinels of orthodoxy who had their own scores to settle with the reformer Sakharam. They would not let Dadaji and Narayan Dhurmaji retreat for fear of Sakharam's formidable position. As Rukhmabai put it, Narayan Dhurmaji and Dadaji, who were acting 'in the hope of getting my little money', were egged on by 'the leaders of our caste' and by 'wicked people (very common in India)'.[5]

A two-pronged offensive was directed against Sakharam to force him to capitulate. He was flooded with offensive anonymous letters, charging him with unjustly 'harbouring' Rukhmabai against the wishes of her husband, and threatening dire consequences if he did not behave. Sakharam was not cowed. Instead, he summoned Dadaji, rebuked him for writing those communications and demanded a written statement to the effect that there was no truth in the allegations. Sakharam, as a long-time benefactor of Dadaji and his brothers, was confident that Dadaji would give in. He was mistaken. Dadaji angrily denied being the author of the anonymous letters, and refused to sign any statement. Thereupon, Dadaji reported, 'Dr Sakharam lost his temper and left me.'[6]

The other prong of the offensive was the threat of legal proceedings. On 19 March 1884, Dadaji sent through his solicitors, Messrs Chalk and Walker, a letter to Sakharam, asking that 'my wife might be allowed to come and live with me as I thought the probation period had lasted long enough'. This was done, primarily, in the hope, as Rukhmabai explains, that Sakharam, 'afraid of losing his reputation', would give in 'because to have a suit of this kind is considered a greatest disgrace among us Hindoos'.[7]

Sakharam was in a difficult dilemma. He was torn between his resolve to support Rukhmabai and the impossibility of ignoring the pressure of his wife and father-in-law for a compromise. But indefinite dithering was not possible. Nor so an immediate clear-cut decision. So, on 22 March, he sent the following reply to Messrs Chalk and Walker:

Gentlemen,

In reply to yours of the 19th instant, I have to inform you that Rukhmabai, mentioned therein, has not been detained at my house against the wishes or demands of your client, Mr Dadaji Bhikaji. Her stay at my house hitherto has been by the consent of the relatives on both sides, because of the unfortunate circumstances of your client.

I have not the slightest wish to detain her even now, and I shall be rather glad if your client provides her with a suitable house and takes her away, which is however his own look out. He is at liberty, so far as I am concerned, to take her away at any time.

Sakharam's reply was a masterpiece of legal equivocation. Saying both 'yes' and 'no', it gave him time for consultations before deciding what was to be done. The opposite party received the reply on the 24th and, predictably, chose to read it to mean 'yes'. Making sure that no more time was wasted, a team appeared the following day at Sakharam's door and announced that, in response to his letter, it had come to take Rukhmabai to Dadaji. The team comprised Narayan Dhurmaji, Damodar Bhikaji (Dadaji's elder brother) and Ganpatrao Raoji, a clerk from the firm of Dadaji's solicitors.

Having in the intervening three days decided not to give in, Sakharam reminded the visiting team of the same letter to say that Rukhmabai could not be sent in the absence of a suitable house and maintenance. Further, this time it was clearly spelt out that suitable house meant 'separate lodging', not Narayan Dhurmaji's house which Dadaji misleadingly called his 'family-house' and 'family residence'.

The very next day, 26 March, a letter was sent on behalf of Dadaji asking Rukhmabai 'to join him forthwith'. She was assured that he would 'give her suitable maintenance and lodging according to his rank and position'. Legal equivocation was now in full play. What Rukhmabai had asked for by way of suitable lodging and maintenance was very different from that which Dadaji promptly promised to give 'according to his rank and position'.

A mere four days of lightning moves by the other party ruled out any more dithering by Sakharam. He had to choose between litigation and condemning Rukhmabai to Dadaji and his surroundings. He was man enough to choose litigation. Once he had resolved upon this course of action, he set out to make the best possible arrangement. He entrusted the case to Messrs Payne, Gilbert and Sayani, a reputed firm of solicitors. The defence was based on the following grounds:

1. The entire inability of the plaintiff to provide for the proper residence and maintenance of himself and his wife.
2. The state of the plaintiff's health in consequence of his suffering frequently from asthma and other symptoms of consumption.
3. The character of the person under whose protection the plaintiff was and is living in the house in which the plaintiff called on the defendant to join him.[8]

Then, in her written submission to the High Court in July 1884, Rukhmabai submitted that she could not be considered bound to the marriage under which Dadaji was claiming the restitution of his conjugal rights. This marriage was solemnized before she had 'arrived at years of discretion', i.e., before she was capable of giving intelligent consent to the marriage. This was a significant move that elevated Rukhmabai's defence to one of high principle. Her case no longer related to specific issues on the settlement of which she would agree to join her husband. It became one of principled refusal to cohabit with him.

Submitting that these were 'the only true reasons for her refusing to live with the plaintiff', Rukhmabai prayed that the case be 'dismissed, and that her costs be provided for'.

That, indeed, was the truth. Rukhmabai had, at last, declared that she was done with this incorrigible man to whom she had been saddled. And also given the reasons why.

This was radical. Not her refusal to cohabit with the man she was married to, but her refusal to recognize the marriage itself. She was but one of the many women who refused to live with their husbands. She was the only one to disown the relationship. In doing this, and in providing a principled justification for the act, she had set an example for the others. An ideal to be fulfilled in reality.

Rukhmabai had heralded a new conception of woman as a person.

Rukhmabai's plea, expectedly, was seen as outrageous. It threatened the very basis on which rested the two pivotal institutions of Hindu society: Hindu marriage and the joint family. Early marriage was then the norm among Hindus, and it was an arrangement between two families. To claim the right to disown one's marriage on the ground of absence of intelligent consent was pure subversion. If recognized, the right would expose every child marriage to the potential risk of being disowned by a spouse after attaining the age of discretion. Recognition of the right to suitable lodging would jeopardize the institution of the joint family.

Rukhmabai's radical plea before the High Court soon found elaborate articulation in the letters of 'A Hindu Lady'. This is evidence enough that the plea was not entirely the work of the solicitors. It was, demonstrably, the plea of a woman who, having as a child taken seven steps with a stranger and seen him 'go through every course of dissipation' in subsequent years, had finally resolved to undo those fatal steps.

It is a measure of Rukhmabai's heightened sensitivity and awareness that she did not resolve upon that extraordinary action because her sufferings were extraordinary. If anything, she was relatively better off than most of her suffering sisters. Yet, it was she who rose up, and offered a resistance that had not been conceived of before.

Revolutions are often initiated not by the poorest and the worst oppressed within a system, but by the relatively better off among them.

Rukhmabai's resolve overrode even her fear of appearing in a law court. When they first met, Rukhmabai nervously asked Nora Scott: 'Must a woman go herself into the court if she has a suit?'[9] Dadaji had already filed the case. She was hoping that the judge's wife might suggest a way to avoid personal appearance. Rukhmabai's fear was part of the general dread that respectable middle-class people had of law courts. Officials and lawyers apart, law courts were not meant for such middle-class folks, certainly not for their women.

Rukhmabai was fortunate that her case came up before a judge, Justice Robert Hill Pinhey, who was sensitive enough to grant her exemption from physical appearance. Other judges would be different.

On 16 April 1885 Sakharam died. For Rukhmabai that was a crippling blow. *Dadaji Bhikaji vs Rukhmabai* had been filed a year ago, but had not yet come up for hearing. And she had lost her lone rock of support in the family. Their notion of family honour and dread of litigation intact, Jayantibai and Harishchandra were unlikely to back her. The case might be dropped before it had really begun.

Rukhmabai now had to protect herself from her mother and maternal grandfather. She had to try and shake them out of their traditional thinking. Time was running out. The case could be listed for hearing any day. The only saving grace was that outside of the family there were well-wishers like Edith Pechey who would not let Rukhmabai despair.

She succeeded. The mother no more demurred; and, even though he could not quite step into Sakharam's shoes, the grandfather decided to take up the unfortunate granddaughter's cause.

Rukhmabai was lucky that her resistance coincided with another event of great public importance. Within months of the filing of *Dadaji Bhikaji vs Rukhmabai*, Behramji Malabari initiated with his celebrated 'Notes on Infant Marriage and Enforced Widowhood' the movement that would eventuate in the epochal Age of Consent Act. Just as he commenced his campaign for legislation, Malabari was advised to collect a few 'test decisions' by courts of law. That would demonstrate the inadequacy of existing laws and the need for fresh effective legislation. Precisely when Malabari received this advice he stumbled upon Rukhmabai's case. The coincidence was a godsend for both Rukhmabai and Malabari.

A master strategist, Malabari was quick to grasp that *Dadaji Bhikaji vs Rukhmabai* alone would establish the urgency of fresh legislation. With his deep identification with women – 'I am the widow,' he famously said – his knowledge of society, politics and history, his powerful pen and caustic wit, he would emerge, through his weekly, the *Indian Spectator*, as the most powerful public voice on the case. He would also work behind the scenes to gather organizational support and funds for Rukhmabai.

Around the same time, Henry Curwen (1845–92) also came over to Rukhmabai's cause. An accomplished writer, Curwen wielded enormous influence as the editor of the *Times of India*. He ensured elaborate pro-Rukhmabai coverage of the case. And before that, he devised a brilliant plan to create an atmosphere in favour of Rukhmabai. He got her to write the letters of 'A Hindu Lady' which we have followed at length in the previous chapter. He encouraged her to write freely and without worrying about space. In an extraordinary move, Curwen inserted editorials that exhorted the readers to read and reflect on the letters.

The timing of the letters was planned with great tactical acumen. The first letter was published in the wake of Malabari's 'Notes', and it began with an appreciative mention of them. The idea was to heighten the effect of the 'Notes' by supplementing them with the searing testimony of a woman. The letter created an air of suspense and expectancy. Who was this mysterious 'Hindu Lady'? What would she say in her next letter? When would that be?

The second letter was even more brilliantly timed. It was published the day *Dadaji Bhikaji vs Rukhmabai* came up for hearing. It made sure that the judge – Mr Justice Pinhey – would have read the piquant exhortation of 'A Hindu Lady' before hearing Rukhmabai's case. He would not miss the uncanny similarity between the two unfortunate women. That, indeed, is how it went. The timing also ensured a similar sympathetic response among the thousands of readers of the *Times of India*. Their response to the shocking revelations in the young helpless woman's case was so much the sharper for having read the previous day's lament of 'A Hindu Lady'.

The plan aroused no immediate suspicion. Subsequently, however, Hindu orthodoxy, wised up by Bal Gangadhar Tilak, complained that this was a conspiracy to put the judge under psychological pressure.

Curwen reminds one perforce of Grattan Geary. We have met him in the first chapter where we had a glimpse of his thorough exposure of Narayan Dhurmaji. Geary was the editor of the *Times of India* when Curwen, freshly arrived from London in 1876, joined the paper as his deputy. Within four years Curwen managed a coup and replaced Geary, who in turn took up the editorship of the *Bombay Gazette*, the city's oldest newspaper. Their rivalry became so intense and public that people avoided inviting both of them to the same function. For an entire decade the rivalry provided colour and verve to Bombay's public life, before ending with Curwen's death in 1892.

Compared to Curwen, Geary was late in throwing his weight behind Rukhmabai. In fact, his first response to her – to 'A Hindu Lady' rather – was critical. Ever ready to support a good cause, Geary hated political correctness. He knew the miseries of upper-caste women. But he also knew that widowhood was not universally 'enforced' in India. Lower-caste women, who formed 'the bulk of the community in the mofussil', laboured under no such disability. Indeed, as one whose own widowed mother had remarried, Rukhmabai should have known that, and refrained from portraying widowhood as a universal practice among Hindus. Citing ample evidence, it was on this ground that Geary faulted 'A Hindu Lady'.

But Geary became an ardent supporter of Rukhmabai from the moment her case came up for hearing in 1885. The following year, when it became clear that the case would drag on and cost a fortune, he even started a fund to help Rukhmabai, who had it immediately closed. Later on, when the Rukhmabai Defence Committee was formed, Mrs Geary became its member. So unqualified was Geary's support to Rukhmabai that he was even dragged in a contempt case by Narayan Dhurmaji.

Such was the power of Rukhmabai's cause that both the arch-rivals, Curwen and Geary, supported her enthusiastically. Only towards the fag end would Curwen cave in.

The stage was ready for a great judicial drama. Initially it was decided that Rukhmabai would be represented by two legal luminaries, Kashinath Trymbak Telang and John Duncan Inverarity, with both of whom Sakharam was on friendly terms. Both he and Telang were prominent public figures who shared a deep commitment to social reform and educational projects. Inverarity, by far the most sought after barrister of the Bombay High Court, was among the earliest and most enthusiastic members of the Bombay Natural History Society, of which Sakharam was a founding member.

A third legal luminary was later added to the team. This was F. L. Latham, the Advocate General of Bombay.

It was not that just any three stalwarts were randomly got together to defend Rukhmabai. The choice of these three was based on a meticulous consideration of the peculiar nature and complexities of the case. Rukhmabai's defence, we have seen, had initially rested on the specific merits of the case, viz., the husband's poverty, ignorance, chronic ill health, and the disreputable surroundings in which he lived. But very soon – raising it to an altogether different plane – it came to rest primarily on certain basic principles of jurisprudence and civilized living. Still later, it would rest exclusively on principles. In invoking these principles, her defence questioned the received mode of judicial thinking and proposed a radical interpretation of the existing laws and legal precedents. Such a daring defence required an outstanding grasp of the intricacies and principles of both English and Hindu laws – the two unequal fountainheads of Anglo-Indian jurisprudence – and a flair for innovative interpretation.

This called for a team of variously gifted and mutually complementing brilliant counsel. It was decided that – to the extent such division of labour was practicable in the courtroom – Inverarity and Latham would conduct the arguments relating to English jurisprudence, and Telang would handle that part of the defence which related to Hindu law.

Telang was particularly qualified to do this. Contrary to the reigning view that Hindu customs and laws were static and regressive, he maintained that they were intrinsically dynamic. It was British rule that 'had stopped the natural and progressive development of

Hindu civilization and had fossilized the law, which but for that would have developed naturally'. The governing principle of Hindu jurisprudence, Telang maintained, was: What custom has made, custom can also ameliorate.[10] Telang would argue that Rukhmabai was a victim of the British Indian judicial system. He would invoke Hindu law to save her.

Dadaji was represented by Vikaji and Mankar. His side obviously believed their case to be so open-and-shut that they saw no danger in hiring two nondescript counsel to counter Rukhmabai's formidable team. It, indeed, proved to be an open-and-shut case in Justice Pinhey's court. But for Rukhmabai.

The case was initially expected to come before Justice Scott. That, in fact, obliged the judge's wife, Nora Scott, to avoid meeting Rukhmabai despite the liking and sympathy she had developed for the brave Hindu girl. In the event, the case came up before Justice Pinhey. That was on 19 September 1885.

$$4$$

Rukhmabai Triumphs

19 September 1885, when dadaji *Bhikaji vs Rukhmabai* came up for hearing, was a Saturday. The High Courts used to work six days a week in those days. Latham, speaking for Rukhmabai, initiated the proceedings before Mr Justice Pinhey. Questioning the very basis of Dadaji's claim, he asked: 'Whether the plaintiff was entitled to maintain the suit?' If the court believed him to be so entitled, two issues would arise. First, 'Whether the plaintiff was in a position to provide for the lodging and maintenance of the defendant', and second, 'Whether the plaintiff was entitled to the relief claimed, or any part thereof'.

Latham did not at this stage raise the issues of Dadaji's health and the questionable character of the man to whose house Dadaji was inviting Rukhmabai to commence the couple's cohabitation. However, if those allegations were proved, Latham reserved the right to avail of them in his client's defence.

Dadaji's counsel countered that the allegations against his client were false. But even if they were true, Hindu law did not entitle Rukhmabai to deny him his conjugal rights. Both the parties to the suit had admitted the fact of their marriage. The onus was now on Rukhmabai 'to prove that she is legally justified in resisting the husband's suit for enforcing his marital rights'. She could not do this on the ground that she had not consented to the marriage. For, as Mayne's authoritative *Hindu Law* made clear, a spouse's consent was immaterial to the validity of marriage. A Hindu marriage, famously, was 'not a contract strictly so called, but a religious duty'.

The stress on the sacramental nature of Hindu marriage was crucial to Dadaji's claim. It showed how he was entitled to the relief he claimed. It could also be used as a possible safeguard against any attempt to so limit the meaning of 'restitution' as to preclude 'institution' of conjugal rights. Marriage was instituted – became binding – the moment the prescribed sacrament was performed. That apart, Dadaji's counsel, paraphrasing Mayne freely, argued:

> From the moment of marriage the Hindu husband is his wife's legal guardian, even though she be an infant, and has an immediate right to require her to live with him in the same house as she has attained puberty; her home is necessarily her husband's home ... Dr Sakharam's house, where the plaintiff frequently visited her, was constructively her husband's place of abode, or, at least, it was a place appointed by him for the purpose of her residence.

Not sure as to how the judge might interpret 'restitution', the counsel prayed, 'in the alternative, for a restitution or institution of conjugal rights'.

Anticipating another argument against the admissibility of Dadaji's claim, his counsel further maintained that there was 'the authority of law texts and the decisions of Courts for holding that a suit for restitution of conjugal rights does lie among the Hindus'.

Regarding the issue of whether Dadaji had the means to provide lodging and maintenance to his wife, Dadaji's counsel contended that the onus of proof lay with Rukhmabai. Nonetheless, they disposed of the issue in principle by maintaining:

The poverty of the husband does not constitute a matrimonial offence so as to operate as a legal bar to the husband's right to seek his wife's society and assistance.

Pinhey did not accept the contention that a suit for restitution of conjugal rights 'would lie between Hindus'. He observed:

I don't agree with Mr Mayne's position, which seems to me to be too broadly laid down by him, and to go much beyond the decisions of the Courts ... the plaintiff must prove his case, and is, therefore, bound to begin.

Evidence was then offered for the plaintiff to prove his case. Two medical practitioners, Dr Gopal Sewram and Dr Vithul Pandurang, testified that there was no basis to the charge that for years Dadaji had suffered from consumption and asthma. Dr Sewram told the court:

I examined plaintiff yesterday and found the lungs quite clear. The bronchial tubes are not affected. I treated him about two weeks ago. I should call him a robust man.

Dr Pandurang was less assertive and more guarded as he told the court:

Plaintiff has no consumptive tendency; at least none is manifest at present. I have examined his lungs since the attack of pneumonia. They are a little weak, owing to his getting a recent cold.

Later in the day, in a testimony that helped the judge make up his mind on the issue of the plaintiff's health, Dadaji's own brother admitted in his deposition: 'Plaintiff's health has deteriorated for some years past.'

The two star witnesses whose evidence was taken that day were Dadaji himself and his uncle, the master plotter, Narayan Dhurmaji. Their testimony related primarily to the plaintiff's material circumstances and his ability to provide lodging and maintenance to his wife. Dadaji testified:

Besides my uncle, during the last year I earned no money from any one except Rs 2 or 4 for preparing plans. I did work for Narayen Wittoba, and he paid me Rs 5. This was the largest sum I got from an outsider.

The total payment he received from outsiders failed to touch double digits. From working for his uncle, however, he claimed to make between five to six hundred rupees every year. When asked to produce documentary evidence for the claim, he answered that he had not kept any papers.

The uncle, in his evidence, said that he paid the nephew between 450 and 500 rupees annually for superintending the work of brick-layers, carpenters and labourers. Asked to produce documentary evidence, he, too, answered that he had kept no accounts, made no entries and taken no receipts.

Justice Pinhey was not impressed. He observed:

The plaintiff gave much false evidence as to his pecuniary position, and his uncle, who was examined on plaintiff's behalf on the same point, gave, if possible, evidence less credible still.

That entire day had been very trying for Pinhey. It had begun at home with him reading the editorial in the *Times of India* and the letter of 'A Hindu Lady'. Little would he have suspected in this a rehearsal of the distressing drama that was soon to be enacted in his court. The distress was overpowering. That night and the following day, he agonized over the thought of having to force that bright, blameless lass into cohabitation with that brute of a husband in the house of his disreputable uncle.

Pinhey wistfully thought of the early 1850s when he had joined service during the rule of the East India Company. He would not then have been saddled with a case such as this, for it was accepted that suits for restitution of conjugal rights had 'no foundation in Hindu law'. He regretted that, following the massive post-1857 restructuring, this peculiar English legal practice had been made part of the British Indian legal regime. A formidable body of case law had since developed. However much he might disapprove of it, he was bound by that case law.

What piqued Pinhey most was the irony that while he, as a judge in British India, was obliged to administer the old cruel English law of restitution of conjugal rights, that law had been humanized the previous year in England.

Pinhey was clear about what he ought to do in the case. But the law hampered him. The only way to escape doing what he knew was barbarous, cruel and revolting was to come up with a legal basis for his decision. Luckily he had an entire Sunday to wrestle with the challenge.

When he left for work on Monday, Pinhey was ready with a judgment in accordance with his conscience. He had had his moment of epiphany. He did not now even need to hear Rukhmabai's defence. So, as soon as Latham got up to speak, Pinhey said:

> Mr Advocate-General, unless you are particularly anxious to make some remarks for the assistance of the Court, I think I need not trouble you as I am prepared to dispose of the case at once.

The message was loud and clear. Latham was promptly back in his seat. Everyone in the courtroom knew something special was coming. They were treated to an inspired judgment at once sagacious and impassioned, morally charged and legally sustainable.

Pinhey pronounced his verdict straightaway. He had 'arrived at the opinion that the plaintiff cannot maintain this action'. He had looked 'into the authorities' – the law as well as the practice of the courts in India and England – and come to the conclusion: 'It is a misnomer to call this a suit for the restitution of conjugal rights.' For:

The parties to the present suit went through the religious ceremony of marriage eleven years ago when the defendant was a child of eleven years of age. They have never cohabited. And now that the defendant is a woman of twenty-two, the plaintiff asks the Court to compel her to go to his house, that he may complete his contract with her by consummating the marriage. The defendant, being now of full age, objects to allowing him to consummate the marriage, objects to ratifying and completing the contract entered into on her behalf by her guardians while she was yet of tender age.

Pinhey was convinced that:

... it would be a barbarous, a cruel, a revolting thing to do to compel a young lady under those circumstances to go to a man whom she dislikes, in order that he may cohabit with her against her will.

The plaintiff would not be justified in 'maintaining the present suit' nor the judge in 'making such an order'.

Pinhey had looked 'into the authorities' to settle the pivotal issue whether a court of law had ever ordered a married woman to go to her husband and allowed 'that man to consummate the marriage against her will'. No court of law, happily, had ever done that. Never

ever had *commencement* of cohabitation, as distinguished from its *resumption* – restitution – been judicially ordered. There was, clearly, 'neither precedent nor authority' to bind him – the judge – to so read restitution as to mean institution. The judge had the discretion to read it either way.

It was no ordinary discretion that Pinhey had excavated from the case law. He had armed the judges – those who cared – with the authority to fuse together law and morality. He could – indeed would – so use the discretion as to *not* do what he believed was barbarous, cruel and revolting. Conjugal rights had not been instituted in the case brought before him. Sure enough, Dadaji had prayed 'in the alternative, for a restitution or institution of conjugal rights'. But, with the discretion he had excavated, Pinhey was free to decide whether he would accept or refuse the prayer. His discretion bound him to refuse:

> especially when the granting of the relief prayed [institution of conjugal rights] would produce consequences revolting not only to civilized persons, but even to untutored human beings possessed of ordinary delicacy of feeling.

Explaining why, he observed with unrestrained candour:

> I am certainly not disposed to make a precedent, or to extend the practice of the Court in respect of suits of this nature beyond the point for which I find authority. The defendant has not appeared in Court, but the evidence shows that she has been brought up in the enlightened and cultivated home of her step-father, the late much-lamented Dr. Sakharam Arjun, a well-known citizen of Bombay. I am glad, therefore, that, in the view of the law which I take, I am not obliged to grant the plaintiff the relief which he seeks, and to compel this young lady of twenty-two to go to the house of the plaintiff in

order that he may consummate the marriage arranged for her during her helpless infancy.

The case, Pinhey ruled, did not lie in law. He dismissed it and awarded costs to Rukhmabai. However, sensing that, Hindu society being what it was, there was a risk of his judgment being misunderstood or misrepresented, he took care to clarify:

Before concluding my remarks I wish to guard myself from being supposed to endorse the contention in the written statement, that the plaintiff was not entitled to claim the society of his wife because he is poor ... A poor man has as much right to claim his wife as a rich man to claim his ... The poverty of the plaintiff is not one of the reasons which I should give for the rejection of plaintiff's claim.

Just when the case seemed over, a veritable explosion occurred. Objecting to the award of costs to Rukhmabai, Vicaji, Dadaji's counsel, submitted 'that this is not a case in which the plaintiff should be ordered to pay costs. He has been acting under advice of counsel who considered the suit would lie.'

In his judgment Pinhey had kept his moral outrage under reasonable restraint. And he had avoided saying the worst that he thought of the plaintiff. Vicaji's request caused him to burst out:

When the plaintiff found that the young lady was unwilling to share his home, he should not have tried to recover her person as if she had been a horse or a bullock.

Nearly twenty years before Pinhey gave vent to his moral outrage against the way women were viewed and treated, Justice Jackson, another British Indian judge had expressed similar sentiments:

A wife cannot be looked upon as property, movable or immovable, which passively undergoes transfer from one person to another. If she could be so dealt with, it would have to be determined whether she was movable or immovable, and some curious questions of limitation might arise; and if the wife were property, she could not, obviously, be a party to the suit, as she is in this, and always must be in suits of this nature. And further, it seems to be repugnant to the principles of civilised society, whether European or British Indian, that an adult human being, wife or otherwise, should be delivered over as a horse or other brute animal might be.[1]

Pinhey's judgment in *Dadaji Bhikaji vs Rukhmabai* was his swansong. His parting gift to India – the land of his birth – and her women. Following indications from the authorities that he was no more wanted, he retired the following month and returned 'home'. He had been a judge of the Bombay High Court for twelve years. All those years he had been known as a weak judge. How could this weak judge make a glorious judicial intervention such as this? Where did his inspiration come from?

The judgment was set off by a lucky convergence of moral sensibility between the litigant and the judge. Rukhmabai was more than a beneficiary of Pinhey's judgment. She was also its catalyst. Here was a young woman who would not submit to the tyranny of custom. She would rather be treated as a person, not a horse or a bullock. She had come to the law to obtain justice. Chance so had it that her case was listed before Pinhey, a judge who, like Justice Jackson two decades earlier, was exceptional in his conviction that law must subserve, not subvert, justice. Failure to save this young woman from custom's tyranny, he recognized, would turn the law into an instrument of torture. Torture not for her alone, but for millions of her similarly victimized sisters. He had the will and the acumen to wrestle with the law to give her justice.

Most judges, not only those known to be weak, would have acted differently. For, they would not have felt impelled to do justice. Judges, as a matter of course, were schooled – and still are – to believe that their job, even as they swore by justice, was to administer the law. They were – and continue to be – trained to take in their stride any miscarriage of justice they might cause in the act of administering the law.

But Pinhey was his own man. It just so happened that he did not feel obliged to do anything judicially spectacular because the normal run of litigation did not involve any serious conflict between law and justice. Hence his reputation as a weak judge, though that should not have been so. For, there was at least one instance, prior to *Dadaji Bhikaji vs Rukhmabai*, in which he had done something unusual. Sitting on a Division Bench, he was cited a Full Bench ruling which he found unacceptable. He disregarded that ruling, saying that 'ten wrongs do not make a right'. No less reflective of his heart and his values is the fact that until his death in 1896 he devoted his post-retirement years to peace work in Europe.

Rukhmabai was really lucky that her case came before Pinhey. But, then, Pinhey could not have delivered his revolutionary judgment if, like millions of her sisters, Rukhmabai, too, had let herself be sacrificed at the altar of custom. Rukhmabai's defiance and Pinhey's conscience had to converge for that revolutionary judgment to be possible. Sadly, though, unlike Rukhmabai, who has been installed where she belongs in history, Pinhey remains unsung and unremembered. The annals of women's emancipation and of Indian judiciary will be fuller and so much more inspiring for remembering him.

5

The Magic of Moral Defiance

RUKHMABAI WAS AN INCONSEQUENTIAL ANONYMOUS litigant on Monday, 21 September 1885, as she waited agonizingly for the evening, when news would reach her of the day's proceedings in her case. The judge had, thankfully, granted her exemption from personal appearance in the court that she had so dreaded. But staying back that day felt no less dreadful. Time hung heavy and the evening seemed painfully far.

Dadaji's plea and his witnesses having already been heard the previous Saturday, that day's hearing was going to be critical. So much would depend on how convincingly her counsel presented her defence. Saturday's proceedings, especially the self-defeating testimony of Dadaji and his key witnesses, had, indeed, provided a ray of hope. But that was just the beginning. The case could take unexpected twists and turns as it unfolded in the days to come.

The news that reached Rukhmabai – well before the evening – was beyond her wildest dreams. She had won. She had won without a word spoken for her. She was a free woman. Rid of her worst fears, she could now turn to the dreams she had dreamt. For the first time in a long time, she could sleep unharassed by evil presentiments.

The following day, 22 September 1885, the anonymous litigant woke up to find herself a celebrity. A celebrity at twenty-two (following Pinhey's verdict). Lionized, overnight, as the champion par excellence of 'the rights of Indian womanhood'.[1] As one who, while the others meekly submitted, had refused 'to be sacrificed' and 'fought the battle, not merely for herself, but also for millions of her sisters'.[2]

Pinhey in his judgment had projected Rukhmabai as an uncommonly cultured and accomplished young lady. That she also possessed uncommon courage was evident from the battle she had fought. The aura her triumph gave her was augmented by the *Bombay Chronicle*'s disclosure that she was the author of the brilliant letters which had appeared under the pseudonym 'A Hindu Lady'.

Ironically, though not unexpectedly, the very circumstance that turned her into an instant celebrity also turned her into an instant villain. Hindu orthodoxy denounced her as a self-centred, wilful woman whose head had been swollen by English education. Aided by a misguided English judge, she had caused a 'revolution' that was 'entirely subversive of the principles that have governed [Hindu] society for ages'. She had brought about an alarming situation in which 'any Hindu wife' could 'any day refuse to go to her husband' with a mere declaration that 'she dislikes him'.[3]

The leaders of Hindu orthodoxy were quick to realize that they had to intervene fast to save their society and culture – their collective being – from subversion. They had to have the misguided judge's decision reversed. Dadaji and Narayan Dhurmaji could not be left alone to decide whether it was worth their while to go in for appeal. Dadaji's case would henceforth be fought by Hindu orthodoxy. Rukhmabai's fight was no longer against her nondescript husband and his scheming uncle. She was now pitted against the Hindu orthodoxy's limitless resources and ruthlessness.

This, in the event, proved decisive. More than is commonly realized, judicial decisions tend to be subtly – even flagrantly – swayed by reigning public opinion. In colonial India this was particularly so. The rulers were wary of alienating entrenched conservative sentiments.

With Hindu orthodoxy threatening dire consequences if its anxieties were not heeded, the outcome of the appeal against Pinhey's judgment was all but certain. Extrajudicial forces had made it a no-win situation for Rukhmabai.

Foremost among those who orchestrated the move to plot Rukhmabai's defeat was Vishwanath Narayan Mandlik (1833–99). A pleader renowned for his practical legal acumen and sound understanding of both Hindu and English jurisprudence, Mandlik had emerged as a powerful voice in public life through his Anglo-Marathi weekly, *Native Opinion*. It was in recognition of his importance that he was, in 1884, nominated to the Viceroy's Legislative Council. Quickest, perhaps, to grasp the gravity of the danger to the traditional Hindu social structure from Pinhey's judgment, Mandlik lost no time to broadcast it through *Native Opinion*. He also assured that it would not be difficult to successfully challenge the judgment, and showed how.

What Mandlik and his *Native Opinion* did in Bombay was done in Poona, the nerve centre of Hindu orthodoxy in western India, by Bal Gangadhar Tilak and his two weeklies, the English *Mahratta* and the Marathi *Kesari*. They did not even mind being vulgar in denigrating Rukhmabai and projecting her as the very picture of what a good Hindu woman would never want to be.

The hysteria generated in Maharashtra travelled far and wide. Suddenly, Hindu orthodoxy all over was bound together in common alarm.

Rukhmabai, too, received a fair degree of public support and sympathy. Virtually the entire Anglo-Indian press – which boasted dailies like the *Times of India, Statesman, Pioneer*, and the *Civil and Military Gazette* – wrote fervently in her favour. In Britain the redoubtable London *Times* made Rukhmabai's cause its own. It provided regular coverage to her case, wrote editorials on it and generously offered its 'Letters' columns for the advocacy of her cause. Some of the most eminent personalities of the day, such as Max Mueller and Bishop Carlisle, used the *Times*' hospitality to highlight the historic significance of Rukhmabai's struggle. A veritable wave of sympathy for Rukhmabai soon swept through England, Scotland, Ireland and Wales. There was hardly a British newspaper or magazine, no matter how insignificant or established, that did not write glowingly of Rukhmabai.

The women of the British Isles felt particularly drawn to Rukhmabai. They sympathized with her as a fellow victim and admired her exemplary struggle. A hundred Scottish women sent a letter expressing their 'hearty co-operation' with Rukhmabai and their other 'Indian sisters who desire to escape from the bondage under which the custom of ages has placed you'. Three Welsh women wrote her a stirring letter, saying: 'You will show what a woman can do, and future ages when women are free and justly treated will bless you as their pioneer. It must be so!' All over there were many more.

No wonder, Rukhmabai's case reverberated even in the House of Commons.

The wave of sympathy and admiration in Britain helped her greatly during the pendency of the case and later on as well. But it also exacerbated the orthodox Hindu perception of threat to their cherished institutions, and strengthened their resolve to thwart the danger.

The appeal against Pinhey's judgment had been planned with great care. Knowing that intricate issues of principles relating to both English and Hindu laws would be raised in Rukhmabai's defence by Latham and Telang – Inverarity was absent this time – Dadaji's legal team was strengthened by the inclusion of Macpherson. In fact, one particular intervention by Macpherson would prove decisive during the hearing.

The appeal was heard by Chief Justice Sargent and Justice Bayley on 12 and 18 March 1886, and the judgment given on 2 April. It is tempting to provide a blow-by-blow account of the fascinating expounding of Rukhmabai's grand defence by Latham followed by Telang. For the purpose of this biography, however, it would suffice to recall certain salient points of the proceedings and of the appellate court's judgment.

That will give an idea of what was historically lost when Rukhmabai lost.

The hearing began ominously for Rukhmabai. Macpherson had barely opened his argument, saying that Pinhey's judgment rested on sentiment and was devoid of legality, when Justice Bayley, throwing judicial reticence to the wind, intervened: 'I don't quite understand on what ground the suit was dismissed, although I have read the judgment more than once.' As if echoing Hindu orthodoxy, Bayley observed: 'According to Mr Justice Pinhey's view, if a lady takes, rightly or wrongly, a dislike to a man, there is an end of the matter.' Echoing the judge, Macpherson added: 'And a number of very pernicious results would ensue if Mr Justice Pinhey's view of the question was given effect to.'

Bayley's self-assured dismissal of Pinhey's judgment betrayed a certain predisposition. Bayley displayed it later also. This happened when Latham, showing why the court was bound to exercise discretion in this case, dwelt on the egregious inequality in the hardship that was involved for Rukhmabai as against Dadaji. Before Latham could complete the argument, Bayley interjected that the hardship was equal; both Rukhmabai and Dadaji were 'tied for life'. Bayley, such was his cognitive blindness, could not comprehend Latham's laconic retort: 'No; they are not.' Macpherson, Dadaji's consul-in-chief, had to explain to Bayley: 'The plaintiff can take another wife.' Sargent, the Chief Justice, also chipped in to enlighten his brother judge: 'If the first wife does not live with him, he can get another; and if she is barren, he can take a third wife. It seems to me the Hindoos are better off than the Mahomedans in this respect. (Laughter)'

One half of the appellate bench was all along hostile to Rukhmabai.

Resuming his opening argument, Macpherson made one significant legal point. He questioned Pinhey's ruling – that this was a case of institution, not restitution, of conjugal rights – on the ground that a Hindu marriage does not require consummation to be complete. Sealing the assertion, Macpherson maintained: 'The Court has no discretion.'

Latham chose two key arguments from Pinhey's judgment to build his defence. One, 'a suit for restitution rights does not lie between Hindus'. The other, 'the present case is without precedent'. He defied the counsel for Dadaji to produce a single 'English authority for enforcing the commencement of cohabitation'. Latham also brought in the question of the mode of enforcing a restitution decree. Recalling rulings in landmark judgments by British Indian judges, Latham warned the appellate bench:

… if we were to hold that a Court could enforce the continuous enforcement of conjugal duties by unlimited fine and imprisonment, we should place the law of this country in opposition to the law of the whole civilized world, except the ecclesiastical law of England.

Latham added that the Hindu law was 'no less humane in this matter than that of other civilized countries'. There was no compulsion to subject Indians to 'severer remedies'.

The heartlessness of the people Rukhmabai was pitted against – Dadaji, Narayan Dhurmaji and the proxy orthodox Hindu litigants – is brought to light by the appellate proceedings. To Latham's impassioned plea about the inhumanity of the execution of restitution decrees, Macpherson's instinctive response was: 'Of course, I am not asking for an execution of the decree.' Even as he said this, the thought of those he represented forced him to add in the same breath: 'I don't know what the views of those who instruct me are as to enforcing the decree.' Having ascertained their views and known what he was expected to do, Macpherson asked the judges to decide according to the law. Queried by the Bench about the inhumanity of executing the decree, he chillingly countered: 'But are your lordships concerned with that in any way?'

Latham, citing some trendsetting English judgments, also presented a compelling case to argue that the court was bound to exercise discretion in this suit. He even managed to elicit from the Chief Justice the observation: 'No woman who has not entered the married state with her free consent should be ordered to go to her husband if she does not like it.' This should have given Latham some hope as he submitted: 'A suit like this I may call a discredited suit, and the court will not step one inch beyond what previous courts have done.' That is, the court will exercise its discretion and not order *commencement* of restitution rights under a law covering *resumption* of those rights.

The argument for Rukhmabai was wound up by Telang. Following up on Latham's erudite and morally charged defence, Telang showed that the law relating to restitution of conjugal rights was alien to Hindu law. Relying primarily on the *Vyavahar Mayukh*, the authoritative shastric text which dealt with litigation before the King's Court, Telang maintained that 'the right for restitution by suit either by the husband or the wife was not constituted' in Hindu law. The Bench, therefore, 'ought to uphold' Pinhey's verdict.

Macpherson then rose to wind up the arguments. He reiterated that the court had no discretion in the matter. He concentrated on two major points made by Latham and Telang. One, that a restitution case was a discredited suit. And second, that such a suit was alien to Hindu law. Macpherson dismissed the first objection on the ground that England may have changed its restitution law a year earlier, but the law in British India remained unchanged. Whether it needed to be changed was 'a matter for the Legislature, and not for this Court'. The court was bound to administer the law as it was.

As for the argument that the case was alien to Hindu law, Macpherson conceded that 'if it could be established that this suit is out of harmony altogether with Hindoo law, I daresay it would be very difficult indeed to say that the suit would lie.' Knowing that there was not a single authority he could cite in his favour, Macpherson took recourse to a sleight of logic. He argued that Hindu law 'contains nothing forbidding' a suit for restitution of conjugal rights. There was nothing in Hindu law that forbade the inclusion of institution within restitution.

Dadaji, therefore, was entitled to the company of his wife.

Sargent and Bayley were glad to accept Macpherson's negative logic. Giving short shrift to Latham and Telang's brilliant advocacy – their impeccable exposition of textual and case law and of the principles of equity and justice – the two judges overturned Pinhey's judgment. They ordered the case to be re-tried.

Technically, Sargent and Bayley could not dispense with a re-trial because Rukhmabai's defence had not been presented before Pinhey. In effect, nonetheless, they managed to pronounce a decree – a deferred decree – against Rukhmabai. They overruled all the principles – the absence of Rukhmabai's consent to her marriage, the distinction between institution and restitution of conjugal rights, and the dubious provenance of British Indian courts' jurisdiction in Hindu cases of restitution of conjugal rights – on which rested Rukhmabai's entire defence. The re-trial would be confined to the merits of the case.

Sargent and Bayley, in effect, had ordered a judicial farce meant to deliver Rukhmabai to Dadaji.

The farce was duly enacted eleven months later, on 3 March 1887, in the court of Justice Farran.

Foreknowing that the matter would end in their favour, Hindu orthodoxy, financed by the ever-calculating *shetyas*, did away with the expensive Macpherson this time. The old duo of Vicaji and Mankar were good enough for the consul's nominal role in the farce.

Latham being away in England, Rukhmabai was represented by Inverarity and Telang. Realizing that there was little they could do to alter the course pre-set by the appellate court, Rukhmabai and her consul did not even care to object to the case being tried by Farran who, as a lawyer before his elevation to the Bench, had drafted Dadaji's original plaint. They had no use for technical trivia. Their gaze was fixed elsewhere. After the requisite procedural steps had been gone through before the Bombay High Court, they would take the case to the Privy Council in London. Latham had even made their intention known to the appellate court. Meanwhile, they would maintain a high moral ground which was likely to improve their chances before the Privy Council.

The farce opened with usual solemnity in Farran's court. Vicaji, speaking for Dadaji, recapitulated the facts of the case. The judge then called upon the defence for its evidence. To that Inverarity responded by demonstrating the futility of the exercise. He could, he submitted, produce evidence to corroborate Rukhmabai's contention that she had not consented to the marriage into which she was being dragged. But the appellate court had already invalidated that. He could also prove that Dadaji, who claimed her company, was unhealthy and too poor to maintain her. But that had been 'practically admitted' in the testimony of Dadaji himself and his witnesses in the court of Justice Pinhey.

Rather than attempt any exercise in futility, Inverarity concluded his brief spirited presentation by saying that he would 'content himself with protesting against the decree which the court would no doubt consider it proper to make'.

Their Lordships – Sargent and Bayley – had in their farce assigned

Rukhmabai the role of a foredoomed silent victim. She, instead, came up with an utterly novel form of resistance and frustrated the entire plot. With due deference to the court, she declared that she would not obey its order to go to Dadaji. She would rather submit herself to the maximum penalty admissible under the law: six months' imprisonment and/or forfeiture of property.

She, who dreaded to go to a court of law, was ready to brave six months in jail. She, who would need to fend for herself as a single woman, was ready to forego all her property.

She would not go to that man.

The 'enslaved daughter' – Rukhmabai's collective self-description for India's womanhood – had had an epiphany. No power could keep a free soul in bondage. She would be a free soul. She had glimpsed the power of moral resistance. Anticipating the power of satyagraha before satyagraha was known, she had turned a notoriously no-win situation into a triumph.

That was 1887. Here is a contrast to appreciate Rukhmabai's action. Four years prior to this, Surendranath Banerjea, the fiery male nationalist, was hauled up for contempt of court for writing a spirited article in his weekly, the *Bengalee*. Advised by W. C. Bonnerjee, the eminent lawyer who would two years later become the first president of the Indian National Congress, Surendranath tendered an apology forthwith. The apology, ironically, could not save him from going to jail.

Farran had no option but to complete the farce scripted by the appellate court. Saying that the case was for institution or restitution of conjugal rights, he ordered Rukhmabai to 'go or return' to Dadaji's house within a month, and inform the court of compliance with the decree.

The judge and the rival consul were, or pretended to be, untouched by the grandeur of Rukhmabai's defiance. So at least their immediate conduct showed. They seemed to want her to be taught a lesson for her intransigence. So, when Inverarity asked Farran to reverse his decision about costs, the peeved judge remarked that had Rukhmabai 'expressed her intention of obeying the decree', he would have made Dadaji pay. Similarly, Dadaji's consul refused even the request for advance notice of the despatch of the bailiff to Rukhmabai's house.

The effect in the world outside was electrifying. Rukhmabai's sworn opponents – the leaders of Hindu orthodoxy – were the first to sense the power of her defiance. They were jubilant, and relieved, that they had, in a mere year and a half, got rid of Pinhey's dangerous verdict. But this was not the triumph they had planned. They had meant to crush Rukhmabai in a way that would serve as a deterrent to future Rukhmabais. That had not happened.

Shrewd men of the world, they sensed that the young rebel had brilliantly outmanoeuvred them. Any attempt to execute the court's decree would give her just the chance she wanted. She would court the requisite punishment, emerge as a martyr and make Hindu culture a laughing stock in the entire civilized world.

Even if Rukhmabai chose not to court punishment and appealed against Farran's decree, Hindu orthodoxy would gain nothing. The reversal of Pinhey's judgment had done what they needed. Hindu law had remained unscathed. Further litigation could culminate in an appeal to the Privy Council, which might restore Pinhey's ruling. The orthodox were most keen to avert that danger.

They were keen to make the decree a dead letter. They had used Dadaji as a pawn to serve their cause and brought him tantalizingly close to getting hold of his wife. Now the cause required them to sacrifice the pawn.

The orthodox, shrewd men of the world would not, of course, admit to having been frightened by the young woman. Forced to try and forestall any more litigation, they provided a new fillip to Rukhmabai's character assassination which had begun after Pinhey's verdict. Besides compensating for their supine surrender, that would help create the illusion that the reason for not enforcing the decree was that no respectable man would deign to live with a 'loose' woman like Rukhmabai.

The lead in fanning this pathological fury against Rukhmabai was all along taken by Tilak's powerful weeklies, the *Kesari* and the *Mahratta*. Within three weeks of Pinhey's judgment, on 13 October 1885, the *Kesari* had pruriently alleged that the judge and the lady were *ekaroopa*, one and the same. After Rukhmabai's defiance in Farran's court, the weekly became more vile and vulgar. On 29 March 1887, in a burlesque entitled 'The Final Scene in the Rukhmabai Farce', it portrayed Rukhmabai as a self-indulgent, licentious woman who would rather go to jail than to her lawfully wedded husband. Was such a woman worth living with?

A close second was Dr Kirtikar, the irrepressible England-returned surgeon and self-professed social reformer. Speaking, of all places, at the Bombay Prarthana Samaj, and claiming first-hand knowledge, Kirtikar detailed Rukhmabai's 'roving sensational life'. Denying that she was a champion of women's emancipation, he said:

Rukhmbai is dependent on her well-wishers. Where is her independence? ... Does it constitute a state of freedom to secure the opportunity of living in association with educated European friends instead of an uneducated husband?

Kirtikar topped his innuendo with the question: 'What will happen to her after another ten years?'[4]

In distant Bengal, its most esteemed weekly, the *Hindoo Patriot*, called Rukhmabai a 'golden lady' and 'Girl of the period', and conjured up a titillating description of her daily routine:

... an accomplished young lady who can sing and dance and play on the piano, and whose proper sphere is the ballroom at night, and the Apollo Bunder or the Bandstand at time of the setting sun ...[5]

Facts, when it came to Rukhmabai, succumbed to febrile imagination even in the case of these otherwise educated, cultured and honourable men. Everyone knew that Rukhmabai, unlike Dadaji, could not marry again. That, in Malabari's unforgettable phrase, she could not escape the 'brutal embrace' of her nominal husband.[6] Yet, condemning her as a woman who had been led astray by her beauty and corrupted by Western lifestyle, *Prachar*, an otherwise respectable Bengali monthly, confidently predicted that she would pick a new husband from among the many *vilayati* and 'native' sahebs she had befriended.[7]

Their hearts bleeding for Dadaji, those sadist men chorused in unison: a licentious woman like Rukhmabai was not worth living with. Some even addressed Dadaji directly, like Kirtikar, who advised him to bid Rukhmabai 'a distant good-bye'.

Hindu orthodoxy was unhinged by Rukhmabai.

Even the stolid colonial dispensation was completely taken aback by her defiance. Discreet enquiries confirming that the young lady was 'determined not to obey' the decree, the Bombay government hurried to request the Government of India to forestall the impending crisis. The Viceroy, to whom the request was addressed, was himself no less rattled. The same day as the Bombay government despatched its request, the Viceroy sent the following telegram to his Law Member: 'I hope you are keeping your eye on the Rukhmabai case. It will never do to allow her to be put into prison.'[8]

Burdened with their civilizing mission, the white rulers did not wish to be seen – in India, in their own country and in the wider world – as sending a woman to prison for daring to follow her conscience.

Dufferin understood something else, too, which shows how well he appreciated the real power of Rukhmabai's defiance and the dynamics of its operation. Months after his telegram to his Law Member, he wrote: 'It would be a good thing for the cause if Mrs or

Miss (?) Rukhmabai were sent to prison; but still we must prevent it somehow.'[9]

Dufferin was not alone. Malabari, that ardent champion of women's cause, wrote, even at the risk of sounding cruel to Rukhmabai, that he would rejoice to see her in prison.[10]

Never before had one solitary individual so ruffled the mighty colonial dispensation.

Even before her case became public knowledge, some prominent individuals with humane and liberal sympathies who came to know about it, such as Malabari, Henry Curwen, Edith Pechey and Nora Scott, had become strong supporters of Rukhmabai. Their number multiplied after Pinhey's judgment. After the great defiance in Farran's court, they were filled with a nervous sense of urgency. Rukhmabai had been given one month to comply with the court's decree. They had within that month to do something to avert the danger of her imprisonment.

Some very influential individuals acted post-haste and set up a committee – the Rukhmabai Defence Committee – for the purpose of affording her all the counsel and aid she needed. The moving spirit behind the initiative was Edith Pechey.

Headed by Principal Wordsworth, the committee comprised representatives of every community – Hindu, Muslim, Parsi, Jewish and European – and all the important sectors of public life. Its immediate objective was to prevent Rukhmabai's imprisonment. As a first step it was decided to file an appeal against Farran's judgment. The appeal, it was known, would end in confirming Farran's decree. The committee's plan was to gain time to press the government for remedial legislation and prepare for an appeal to the Privy Council.

On 7 August 1887, the committee sent a memorial to the Government of India. Summing up 'the very painful position' in which Rukhmabai had been placed, the memorialists said:

That her appeal will probably be heard in course of a few days, and
if decided against her, she must, in the event of Dadaji applying to
have the decree enforced, either admit him to full conjugal rights, or
go to prison, or seek further temporary protection by the very costly
process of an appeal to the Privy Council.

Further, because Rukhmabai 'resolutely persists in refusing'
cohabitation, and the proposed legislation to modify the existing law
of restitution of conjugal rights was getting delayed, the memorialists
asked the government 'to take into consideration the extreme
urgency of Rakhmabai's case and pass a short Act suspending the
provisions of the Code [of Civil Procedure] ... so far as they relate
to imprisonment in the case of married persons who have never
cohabited.'

Meanwhile the fury of Rukhmabai's opponents found public
expression in a vicious attack on her. An obviously ghostwritten
statement – most probably from Dr Kirtikar's caustic pen – was
published in Dadaji's name on 11 April 1887. Entitled 'An Exposition
of Some of the Facts of the Case *Dadaji Vs. Rakhmabai*', it appeared
in the *Times of India* on 19 April 1887. Subsequently, it was widely
circulated as a pamphlet.

Rukhmabai was in a quandary. Should she ignore the attack or
issue her defence? After two and a half months of reflection and
consultation with friends, she had her 'Reply' published in the *Times
of India* and the *Bombay Gazette* on 29 June 1887.

Narayan Dhurmaji, whom Rukhmabai had exposed in this 'Reply',
filed a case of libel against her, her grandfather, Harichand Yadowji,
and the editor of the *Bombay Gazette*, Grattan Geary.

The case ended disastrously for Narayan. But it caused Rukhmabai
great vexation. For example, Hemming, Narayan's boorish lawyer,
refused to carry on unless Rukhmabai was physically present in the
courtroom. His sole purpose was to expose her to the lecherous

crowd that had thronged the court to feast on this 'free' woman. The trauma of it for young Rukhmabai, whom the High Court had granted exemption from personal appearance, is evident in what, four agonizing weeks later, she said to the magistrate, Crawley-Boevy. She begged him, in English:

> Those people, that is the opposite party, are doing all those things to bring me into trouble. I ask the protection of the Court and that the case may be proceeded with as rapidly as possible to relieve me from my trouble.

Vexatious though the libel case was, Rukhmabai was lucky that a member of her Defence Committee, the great nationalist leader Pherozeshah Mehta, appeared for the defence along with another big lawyer, James Jardine. Mehta and Jardine capped the savage exposure of Narayan Dhurmaji, the complainant, which Grattan Geary had initiated.

Rukhmabai and her grandfather were fully vindicated as the magistrate remarked:

> She and her grandfather had been bitterly aspersed and maligned in the public prints and in public lectures. They had been held up to public odium and ridicule. They had been publicly challenged by Dadaji to reply to his exposition ... The imputations against Narayan Dhurmaji have, in my opinion, undoubtedly been made by Rukhmabai with due care and attention.[11]

The libel case also proved an unlikely boon for Rukhmabai. Lurid disclosures about Narayan Dhurmaji, to whose house the High Court had ordered Rukhmabai to go to cohabit with Dadaji, offered a preview of the life she was being condemned to. A young woman of culture, people could see, was being judicially forced into the arms of a loafer in the house of a lech. The effect of Rukhmabai's defiance was redoubled by the knowledge of what it was that, come what may, she would not submit to.

Earlier the judges were swayed by Hindu orthodoxy. Now they were also worried about the opposite public opinion. The judges saw wisdom in procrastination and dodged the danger of deciding one way or the other. They let the appeal hang fire. Finally, the matter ended a year later, on 5 March 1888, with a compromise verdict which the rival parties asked the appellate bench to issue along the lines they had agreed on.

This was a carefully drafted compromise that protected Rukhmabai comprehensively from all immediate and future complications. Dadaji received two thousand rupees from Rukhmabai 'in satisfaction of all costs'. He undertook 'not in any way to execute the decree, nor in future to assert any claim by suit or otherwise as a husband against defendant's person, or her present and future estate'.

Rukhmabai was a free woman. Except for the legal bar to marry again, and for the invisible cultural impulses that nestled deep within her and would suddenly surface and possess her years later.

The compromise may seem a let-down. It was definitely a deviation from, if not desertion of, the principles and spirit that had animated Rukhmabai's fight. Seen closely, a very different story emerges. It is possible that the desire for a dignified quiet life following the exhaustion of a mismatched fight was behind Rukhmabai's acceptance of the compromise. If so, she was entitled to be left alone. She could not, after all, be expected to consume herself in an endless fight. But it was something more compelling that led her – against her own instinct and better reason – to accept the compromise.

Precisely when Hindu orthodoxy and the ruling dispensation were conspiring for a compromise, Rukhmabai was beginning to feel disenchanted due to certain unexpected developments. The first setback came from Henry Curwen, the editor of the *Times of India* who, along with Malabari, had from the beginning been a major ally. On 6 July 1887, Narayan Dhurmaji sent the *Bombay Gazette* and the *Times of India* a legal notice, asking them for the original of Rukhmabai's 'Reply' to Dadaji's 'Exposition', which the two dailies had published, or else face libel. The *Times of India* complied tamely. The *Gazette* refused, asserting its right and obligation to protect its informants.

Then, chided by the *Gazette* for letting Rukhmabai down, the *Times of India* replied lamely:

When we published the letters of 'A Hindu Lady', we accepted the fullest responsibility for them, and we were bound to keep her secret. But when Rukhmabai writes to us over her own name, about family squabbles of which we can know nothing, we leave the primary responsibility with her. [12]

Rukhmabai saw through Curwen's dissimulation. It was the truth behind these family squabbles, which he now claimed to know nothing about, that had once prompted him to lend her his unwavering support. She could sense in the *Times of India* a growing cooling off towards her. She had first noticed it in the immediate wake of Farran's order. The *Times of India* had in 1885 complimented Pinhey for doing in the course of a morning's work more for Indian womanhood than had ever been accomplished. But now it pronounced the same verdict to be 'not sound in law' which subsequent benches had done well to reverse.[13]

This was ominous. If an avid supporter like Curwen could as good as leave her mid-stream, what was in store for her, worried Rukhmabai.

An even more crippling blow came around the same time. Following the manner in which Sargent and Bayley had reversed Pinhey's decree, it was plain that the Bombay High Court was for her a blind alley now. All she could gain here was some time. Her only hope lay in an appeal to the Privy Council. But that would materialize only if the Rukhmabai Defence Committee backed her fully like the Hindu orthodoxy had backed Dadaji.

That kind of backing seemed certain when the Defence Committee came into being. Actually the first impression the committee conveyed was that it had resolved upon taking the case to the Privy Council. But, then, one of its most important members, Telang of all persons, put his foot down. Telang had joined the committee on the condition that its efforts would be concentrated on saving Rukhmabai from being imprisoned. Neither the committee nor Telang then realized that serious differences would soon erupt between them about how to achieve that end.

Telang was no run-of-the-mill social reformer. He was seriously concerned about the difficulty of reforming a society under foreign domination, particularly one like the Hindu society which took legitimate pride in its venerable traditions. The Hindus had long been wary of foreign rulers' intervention in their domestic and socio-religious arrangements. Telang wanted the reformers to be sensitive to the Hindus' fears and operate without alienating 'public opinion'. This might take time and necessitate, for the time being, unreasonable concessions to the regnant orthodoxy. Effective social reform could only be a slow, delicate operation.

Rukhmabai's challenge in open court had thrown the already charged Hindus into a kind of mass hysteria. Even greater delicacy, and readiness for compromise, was in the circumstances expected of social reformers. Telang was now not ready to even stick to the line of action – taking the case to the Privy Council – he and Latham had proposed during the hearing before the High Court.

The moment he sensed that the Rukhmabai Defence Committee planned to approach the Privy Council and challenge the validity of Rukhmabai's marriage, Telang shot off a long letter, dated 24 April

1887, to the committee. He would not, he said, countenance any action that raised issues of principle like absence of her consent in the marriage, the distinction between restitution and institution, or the court's jurisdiction in Hindu marriages. He asked the committee not to plan an appeal to the Privy Council.

Telang told the committee that it was being popularly perceived as plotting to destroy the system of early marriage. If it failed to restrain itself, he warned, the committee would arouse the 'irreconcilable opposition' of 'the whole Hindoo community'.

Further, in an offensive that badly disconcerted the Rukhmabai Defence Committee, Telang made his letter public. He sent it to the *Times of India* which, already beginning to cool towards Rukhmabai, the daily happily published on 26 May 1887.

A special meeting of the committee was summoned to discuss the letter. The members had a hard decision to make. They had two options. They could take Rukhmabai's – women's – cause to the bitter judicial end, no matter what the consequences; or they could accept Telang's plea for an amicable solution without foregoing the cause. The discussion that followed was most animated. But it ended with the committee bowing to Telang's pragmatism.

The committee's support to Rukhmabai, obviously, was nothing like the organized Hindu orthodoxy's support to Dadaji. Self-preservation had prompted Hindu orthodoxy to support the latter. The Rukhmabai Defence Committee rhetorically invoked women's cause, but it was content with saving her from punishment and safeguarding her future. It was happy that it had made 'the full provision of the entire expenses' for the trial that had secured her freedom.

What, after this, was Rukhmabai left to fight with? And what for? The compromise was not an offer from Dadaji that she could have peremptorily rejected. It had been engineered behind the scenes by the very powers – Hindu orthodoxy and the Raj – that her defiance had forced to run for cover. They both were desperate to end the matter without losing face. Rukhmabai, in rejecting the compromise, might deny them that chance. The court would, then, have to decide on her appeal against Farran's decree. Everyone knew what that decision would be. What fight would she wage then?

Rejecting the proffered compromise would leave her with two obviously impractical alternatives. She could accept the everyday hell of cohabitation with Dadaji and altogether abandon the cause; or else she could court punishment and become a sacrificial saint, knowing that the sacrifice would not further the women's cause beyond what she had already done.

Rukhmabai was far from happy with the compromise. She would have ideally liked a more edifying end to the four years of her resistance. Her disappointment is evident in the letter she sent to the Defence Committee before leaving for England. After thanking the Committee 'for their consistent and generous help and assistance in my hour of need', she ruefully remarked: 'The objectives that we had kept before the Committee are not fully achieved.'[14]

The compromise continued to hurt Rukhmabai. Her gnawing regret comes alive in an eponymous poem by Catherine Amy Dawson, a young poet who got the entire sad story from Rukhmabai when she was studying medicine in London. She says in the poem:

> … but the men
> Who wrought against us feared the sympathy
> Which would look richly out of English eyes,
> And offered to forego their specious claims
> For a consideration of rupees –
> Red gold in lieu of a reluctant wife.
> And those about me urged the compromise
> I yielded – to repent before the day
> Had gathered in its sheaves of light. The law

Was stayed, but the decisive 'yea' or 'nay'
Which should determine the uncertain fate
Of generations to come, yet remains
A space unspoken.

That grim uncertainty of law makes Rukhmabai rue:

… Better I had borne
The pain of durance – aye, and greater pains –
If by so doing I had roused the world
Into repression of old usages,
Which, cursing the sad mothers of our race,
Recoil upon their children.[15]

Rukhmabai had done her best. It was time she bowed out gracefully.

Her struggle was epochal. It opened up possibilities and promises that generations have since striven to realize. That is the way epochs are shaped. Over generations.

6

Another Brave Decision

RUKHMABAI HAD REASON TO FEEL bad about the whimper with which her struggle ended. But it also taught her a lesson or two about the ways of the world. She learnt that, no matter how hard you aspire, there are limits to the good you can do in one lifetime. She also learnt that when it came to vilifying her, even the respectable felt no qualms. And she learnt to still stand tall.

In any event, though, she was relieved that it was all over. Now she had to equip herself for the life of a self-reliant single woman. Auto-schooling alone would not help. She had to acquire some kind of professional competence. She was nearing twenty when the litigation started. There was little she could do so long as she was trapped in the cares, anxieties and uncertainties of the case. Time was running out. The longer the litigation lasted, the harder it became to start training for something worthwhile.

Seen that way, the litigation did not end a moment too soon. At twenty-four, she needed to decide fast about what she wished to be. Of her three guardians, the one who could have guided her was dead. While he was alive, planning a career for Rukhmabai had not been a matter of concern for Sakharam. Neither Jayantibai nor Harishchandra Yadavji had the breadth of vision to offer her sound advice. For Jayantibai, particularly, it was very difficult to think of a future for her daughter without being constrained by considerations of community, religion and tradition.

It was actually her guardian angel, Edith Pechey, who, by her personal example and gentle guidance, helped Rukhmabai choose her career. She would be a doctor. This choice was in consonance with her aspiration to lead a life of service. It would, besides, ensure her the respectable middle-class status to which she had been used.

The decision that she would train for medicine was made only once the case was over. However, the desire to be a doctor had flitted across her mind after coming close to Edith Pechey. The more the young, impressionable and harassed Rukhmabai learnt of Pechey's life story, the stronger became her urge to emulate the pioneering English woman doctor. Then, sensing the moment to be ripe, in 1886 when Rukhmabai was in the thick of a public storm, Pechey lent her a copy of Sophia Jex-Blake's *Medical Women*. The book's effect was electrifying. Dropping not 'a single word of it', Rukhmabai read fervently through that vivid first-hand account of the trials and tribulations of the brave 'Edinburgh Seven'. Uncertain of how her own fight would end, she gained 'great comfort' from the fact that 'the truth won the victory at last'. It gave Rukhmabai great comfort in the hour of her trial to be with one of those intrepid seven, Pechey.

As she proceeded with *Medical Women*, the desire to be a doctor – for a life of service – began to feel real. It would be incredible to do for her countrywomen what the noble-spirited Englishwoman had come from thousands of miles to do for them. The early stirrings of that desire also made Rukhmabai prone to anxiety and fear. She would worry that her paltry self-education was far too inadequate to qualify her for medical education. Again, it was Pechey who would engage Rukhmabai in long conversations, remove her fears and assure her that she had it in her to be a good doctor.

In normal circumstances it would not have been a difficult decision to implement. Bombay had its own Grant Medical College. Chance so had it that, after having been a male preserve for the first four decades, the college had just five years earlier, in 1883, opened its portals to women. In fact, the first batch of its women doctors came out the very year the Rukhmabai case ended and it was decided that she should be a doctor. Also, Sakharam Arjun had been among the most distinguished alumni of the college and its authorities would have readily accepted his daughter as a student.

But circumstances were not normal. Rukhmabai's case had ended, not the angry hatred against her. Cessation of her character assassination formed no part of the compromise with which the case had come to a close. If anything, having failed to break her through the mechanism of law, the orthodox were set on destroying her by other means. The chief of those means was to reduce her to a miserable everyday existence by projecting her with greater ferocity than before as a woman of easy virtues, creating an atmosphere in which she could not step out without having vulgar remarks and lewd gestures hurled at her. The situation was made even more threatening by the prevailing societal hostility to women who dared to become doctors and, refusing to stay confined within the homes, ventured out as independent professionals.

Risking going to the Grant Medical College in that volatile atmosphere would be insane. It was best for Rukhmabai to be away from the scene. Even though, compared to the Grant Medical College, gaining admission to a medical college in the UK was more difficult and doing a five-year course there very much more expensive, that was the only feasible option.

Pechey had anticipated this at the outset. Rukhmabai tells us that 'all through the four long weary years of my trial ... she [Pechey] constantly urged me to proceed to England and study Medicine'. Pechey had helped Sophia Jex-Blake in the founding of the London School of Medicine for Women. She had served as a member of the School's Governing Body and delivered its prestigious inaugural lecture for 1878. She knew well the Dean of the college, Dr Elizabeth Garrett Anderson, the first female doctor of Britain, as well as some other teachers, especially Dr Isabel Thorne, who was one of the Edinburgh Seven. It would not be difficult for her to get Rukhmabai admitted to the school.

Once Rukhmabai was won over to the idea, Pechey set about realizing it. She persuaded the Rukhmabai Defence Committee to aid, to the extent they could, Rukhmabai's medical education. The committee's contribution was enough to meet her passage to, and initial expenses in, London.

The problem of finances, however, was bigger than that. Rukhmabai would need to spend a minimum of five years in the UK to complete her education. That would cost a great deal. Pechey got in touch with influential individuals and institutions in the UK. Through these contacts she not only obtained adequate funds but also enlisted families and individuals who were willing to look after Rukhmabai during her sojourn.

While making these arrangements Pechey was particularly concerned that Rukhmabai should not face any want that might distract her from her course. Knowing what it was to be a woman in Britain and also that things could be worse for a woman from India, Pechey wanted to make sure that Rukhmabai was placed in an enlightened, liberal and welcoming atmosphere. She was delighted when Eva and William McLaren responded to her call on behalf of Rukhmabai. The McLaren couple were among the most prominent and enthusiastic champions of women's cause. They wrote that they wished to be Rukhmabai's local guardians, adding that she would stay with them for the first year to get used to London before shifting to a hostel.

While acknowledging Pechey's role in the entire enterprise, it must be recognized that her success was in no small measure facilitated by the fact that Rukhmabai's historic struggle had already made her famous in the UK and earned her widespread sympathy.

No less encouraging, but more predictable, was the response of Elizabeth Adelaide Manning who, next only to Mary Carpenter, was perhaps the most eminent of India's British women friends. Manning and the Indian National Association, of which she was the moving spirit, were especially concerned with the question of medical women for India and with the welfare of Indian students in the UK. Besides, she had followed the Rukhmabai suit from the very outset, and the *Journal of the National Indian Association* had, in its issue for September 1885, reproduced the first of her two celebrated letters to the *Times of India* in the form of an article on 'Child Marriage in India'. In fact, Manning happened to be in Bombay prior to Rukhmabai's departure for England. The two met and, to make things easy for Rukhmabai, it was decided that she would take the same ship as Manning.

While making preparations for Rukhmabai's medical education in London, Pechey took care to prepare Rukhmabai for life and study in the UK. She got Rukhmabai to receive special lessons to improve her English, honed her conversational abilities in the language and instructed her in the basics of English habits, manners, customs, etiquette, etc.

Finally, a delicate operation needed to be performed at home before the plan could be implemented. It was certain that Jayantibai and Harishchandra Yadavji would oppose the plan. Their natural protective instincts would not let them even think of abandoning the young girl to be all by herself in a far-off alien land. They would also be held back, no less, by the dread of the social sanctions that would be visited upon them for their ward's violation of the traditional ban on sea voyage. Let us recall Rukhmabai's account of what transpired:

It did not take [Pechey] long to convert me to her views, but the difficulty lay with my mother and grandfather. Even now it is not an easy matter for a Hindu to cross the 'black waters' ... twenty years ago it was almost impossible.[1]

Converting the mother and the grandfather was a difficult operation, and it had to be performed by Rukhmabai all alone. She found herself handicapped in performing it by her inability to allay in their entirety the natural fears and anxieties of her two guardians. She was ready to concede as much as she could without compromising her principles. But they wanted more. So, gently and patiently, she pleaded with them until they gave her their permission and blessings.

The story is typical of what, in such situations, happened in Hindu families in those days. Even as the two guardians veered reluctantly towards letting their girl go, they wanted from her three assurances that would lessen their apprehensions and the burden on their Hindu conscience. They wanted her to promise three things: she would not eat beef; she would not marry an Englishman; and she would not renounce her religion and become a Christian.

Rukhmabai gave the last two assurances readily, but categorically refused to not eat beef. She was clear about her convictions and possessed the courage to act accordingly. It was no easy matter for a Hindu to disregard the taboo on beef. Precisely when she did this, the distinguished savant, Dr Rajendralala Mitra, was under fire for maintaining that beef was eaten in ancient India.

Jayantibai and Harishchandra had the good sense to be content that, no matter what she ate in England, their rebellious girl would return a Hindu unencumbered with an English husband. Nonetheless, that they sought those three assurances shows how little her mother and grandfather knew her. Had they known her, they would have realized the redundancy of seeking the last two promises, if not also the impossibility of extracting the first. With even an inkling of the disgust their girl felt for marriage, they would have rest assured that, not just an Englishman, she would marry none. Similarly, had

they understood the rationale of her uncompromising attack on
the reigning socio-religious evils, they would have realized that she,
nonetheless, remained a Hindu at heart. As for beef, she believed
the revulsion for it to be just one of the Hindus' many superstitions,
which she was not obliged to share.

Clearly, Rukhmabai experienced psychological-emotional
isolation even in a family more open and less constraining than the
average Hindu family of her day.

7

Six Years in England

Rukhmabai left for England on 22 March 1889. That was a fortnight later than her scheduled departure. Elizabeth Adelaide Manning, with whom Rukhmabai was meant to travel, had already left. Travelling alone made the long journey more difficult and less instructive than it would have been in Miss Manning's company. However, moving farther away from home and being still away from her destination gave her plenty of leisure to reflect on her life as it had been and on how she now wished to shape it.

She knew that she had been afforded a great opportunity. She was going to study at Britain's premier medical school for women. That would equip her for the life of service she had long dreamt of. The dream, for the first time, was within her grasp. She was also, at the same time, assailed by doubts: did she have it in her to do it? The fear had seized her earlier, too, and Pechey had helped her get over it.

That was a temporary reprieve. The fear had its roots in her unpreparedness for advanced education. She had been a persevering auto-didact. But that had not repaired the damage done by the denial of formal schooling. She had completed a crash course prior to leaving for England. But that did not make her feel equipped to face the challenge. That confidence would come gradually and with greater effort and time. Indeed, a sense of inadequacy and inferiority would plague her for much of her stay in the UK.

Any student setting out for higher studies abroad would have felt troubled. But the burden Rukhmabai carried was out of the ordinary. She was not an anonymous individual aspirant going out at the family's expense who, if she failed, would cause a personal and familial setback. If she failed, she would fail all those who, trusting her, had sponsored her. She would also fail a large cause. The thought was unbearable, and avoiding it impossible. The long voyage was a ceaseless oscillation between high hopes and deep depression.

It ended on a dismal fog-ridden afternoon. London could not have been less welcoming to the newcomer. If this is what a spring afternoon was like here, how would she, used to the clear temperate air of her native Bombay, last out five years?

Even as she worried about survival, Rukhmabai found herself in the warm embrace of her hostess, Lady Eva McLaren, and her husband Sir Walter McLaren. The couple had driven down to the London Port to receive her. Their house would be Rukhmabai's home for the first year and Eva her local guardian during her studentship.

A Liberal member of the House of Commons, thirty-six-year-old Sir Walter McLaren belonged to a distinguished Scottish Whig family. His father, Duncan McLaren, had been a very influential Liberal MP from Edinburgh, and so were his two elder brothers. John Bright, the famous Radical MP, was Walter's maternal uncle. His mother, Priscilla Bright McLaren, was a leading suffragist and long-serving president of the Edinburgh Society for Women's Suffrage. No surprise that Walter felt drawn to a budding suffragist, Eva Muller, one year his senior, and the two got married. In partnering with his wife to so generously support Rukhmabai, Walter was only following the example of his parents, who had stood up for the 'Edinburgh Seven' and been instrumental in ensuring that women were accepted as medical students at the University of Edinburgh.

Eva, daughter of a German father – a rich businessman – and English mother, was brought up in a liberal domestic atmosphere. Her mother, Maria Henrietta, was a woman of progressive political views. Her elder sister, Henrietta, was a staunch feminist who founded and edited the *Women's Penny Paper*, later named the *Woman's Herald*. (Early in the 1890s Henrietta became a Theosophist and later a follower of Vivekananda.) Eva was but a schoolgirl when, in keeping with her domestic environment, she began her apprenticeship to philanthropic work under the guidance of eminent social reformer Octavia Hill and worked among the urban poor. She also worked with that foremost champion of women's rights, Josephine Butler, during the agitation that brought about the repeal of the Contagious Diseases Act. Eva's marriage with Walter made her the niece, and soon an ardent follower, of Margaret Bright Lucas, a committed suffragist and also the founder of the British Women's Temperance Association. Her experience of working in different fields of social reform convinced Eva that, to be real and lasting, reform must be all-round and universal, not piecemeal.

Despite her holistic understanding, Eva believed that women's right to vote came 'first'. Until 'we get that [the vote],' she argued, 'half the community is eliminated from having a say upon the proposed measures of reform.' Insisting that there must be 'one moral code for men and women alike', she went to the heart of the problem: 'I think it important that women should make a special effort to further the interest of their sex, because men with the very best intentions have not been able to secure those measures which will give to women their best development.'

Eva envisaged 'a united sisterhood upon the wide platform which embraces all those reforms and which stands for "God and home and every Land".'[1]

As one who practised what she believed, and possessed the means to do so, Eva felt inspired to host her suffering, crusading

Indian sister. Eva was not alone. The good deed was actually initiated by her mother, Mrs Muller, with the provision of a sum of 3,500 rupees.[2] Lady Cowasji Jehangir, a member of the Rukhmabai Defence Committee, would recall forty years later that 'we were surprised to receive a letter from Mrs Muller, an English lady, offering her [Rukhmabai] a home'.[3] Eva's sisters, too, pitched in with their contributions.[4] There were also other unnamed ladies who promised to subscribe when further funds were needed.

Rukhmabai's shock on arrival evaporated as she soon discovered how welcoming and generous London – indeed, the UK – was to her. She had not come out to Britain as a mere student. No Indian – not even Raja Rammohan Roy earlier in the century and Pandita Ramabai in Rukhmabai's own day – had been lionized throughout Britain like she was even before she had dreamt of setting foot on British soil; and all through her stay in the UK she was widely welcomed and admiringly written about. That the British saw her as one of their own is indicated in the *Idylls of Womanhood,* a collection of seven poems by Catherine Amy Dawson, a coeval of Rukhmabai who had sought and befriended her. Appearing two years after Rukhmabai's arrival in the country, the book carried a twenty-six-page poem, entitled 'Rukhmabai', providing an intimate and inspiring account of her life. Similarly, a perspicacious American woman settled in the UK wrote: 'There is no more interesting personality from India in England than Rukhmabai ... For myself, I hardly know such a heroine anywhere.'[5]

This exceptional heroine was widely welcomed in the British press. The following excerpt shows how her arrival – obviously following a news agency's release – was typically reported:

Rukhmabai, the Indian lady whose refusal to live with her husband, to whom she had been married when an infant, created so much interest last year and the year before in England and in India, has arrived in this country with a view to entering the Women's Medical

College, and pursuing a course of study there which will enable her to obtain the necessary qualifications to practise medicine. Before leaving India she addressed a farewell letter to the secretary of her defence committee explaining the circumstances under which she leaves that country for a time. After thanking the committee for its constant aid, and expressing a hope that their joint success, though only partial at present, "will go a great way to lessen the miseries of such of my Hindoo sisters as may be unfortunately situated like myself," Rukhmabai states that through the exertions of a lady doctor in India, Mrs Pechey-Phipson, she has obtained a home in this country from Mr M'Laren, M.P., and Mrs M'Laren, who have undertaken to find the funds for her medical education.[6]

Flattering as this was, there was more to make Rukhmabai feel welcome, and at home, in London. From the moment she arrived she began receiving invitations to important functions and events. One of these was to an impressive soiree organized by the National Indian Association on 8 May 1890. Present at the soiree were many distinguished people she had known back home. They included Lord and Lady Reay, who had just returned after the completion of Reay's term as governor of Bombay, Nora Scott, Mr and Mrs Cowasji Jehangir, and Behramji Malabari.

Comforting as it was for Rukhmabai to meet so many familiar people, the most heart-warming was the reunion with Nora Scott. These two women, we will recall, had developed a mutual fondness when they first met at Edith Pechey's in Bombay, but Nora was soon obliged by her husband's judgeship of the Bombay High Court to avoid contact with Rukhmabai. Nora's husband had retired in 1890 and the family had returned home in London around the time Rukhmabai reached there.

Inundated with invitations, Rukhmabai had no chance to feel lonely or overly homesick. As Nora Scott remarked, if 'Rukhmabai had accepted all the invitations from kind friends, and had gone about to parties and amusements, as she could have done, she could not have had time for the hard work that was necessary'.[7]

The esteem in which Rukhmabai was held in the UK is affirmed by the fact that whenever she attended a public function, her name was invariably listed among the dignitaries present on the occasion. All through her six-year sojourn, to quote the distinguished British surgeon Louisa Martindale, Rukhmabai remained 'very much in the limelight'.

But what truly made her feel at home and confident was being with the McLarens. Besides initiating her into the life of the aristocracy, they exposed her to a whole range of new expansive experiences. The McLarens had two houses; one in a secluded street known as the Poet's Corner, adjoining Westminster Abbey and within a hundred yards of the Houses of Parliament, and the other in the affluent London suburb of Maidenhead.

Life for Rukhmabai at the McLarens' turned out to be radically different from what it had been back home. She was assigned a room of her own. She also had hours of the day that belonged exclusively to her. The radicality of the difference did not lie in the McLarens' material circumstances or their notion of hospitality; it lay in the fact that living life that way was for them, and in their society, a matter of principle.

To grasp that radical difference we may recall Rukhmabai's uncomplaining remark to Nora Scott: '[O]ur children never play, you know.' One of the first things the McLarens did was to take this stranger to play on their tennis court. Not to watch but to play tennis. Here is an admirer's gushing description of Rukhmabai within months of her arrival in London. After remarking that there was nothing Rukhmabai's new friends could teach her regarding the social problems of the day, the admirer writes:

Their chief difficulty with her is to teach her to play lawn tennis. It is contrary to caste for a high-caste woman in India ever to run. Not only had Rukhmabai never run a yard herself until she arrived in this island, but none of her ancestresses for countless generations had run a yard either, and she is thus handicapped by a primeval hereditary disability; but what she lacks in freedom of limb is almost made up by quickness of eye and suppleness of wrist.[8]

Tennis would become one of the few joys in the sad life of Rukhmabai.

Her life had not been one of material deprivation. It was not for nothing that Dr Sakharam Arjun, her stepfather, was called the 'Lord', and his house described as palatial. Yet, for all its affluence and high social position, the family's lifestyle was frugal and minimally reliant on paid domestic help. All the major household chores, like cooking and children's care, were performed by the women of the family. Beginning with the birth of her first step-sibling – when she herself was a child – till her departure for England, Rukhmabai had been part of the domestic workforce. Ceaseless pressure of work, combined with social norms, left no room for women's leisure, let alone their privacy. All those years Rukhmabai had pined for a bit of her own space and time, and got none. She had wanted her craving for education to evoke a sympathetic response. It was brushed aside.

At the McLarens she got both as a matter of course. She was filled with an exhilarating sense of liberation. For the first time, she breathed freely. And did so without causing either the family or herself any harm. Contrary to what traditional socialization had drilled into her, Rukhmabai realized that having one's privacy, dignity and freedom was no reason to carry the guilt of selfishness. Individual members' freedom and dignity were essential for a family's happiness, not a hinderance.

This was a life-changing experience. No more would Rukhmabai be the kind of family person she had been conditioned to be. Once back in India, she would not let herself be mired into the affairs of her Bombay-based family. She would return to Bombay after retirement, but not to the bungalow her mother had built. She would live in the house she had built for herself. Maintaining her distance, she would do whatever she felt she should for her step-siblings, their children and grandchildren. Ready for solicited advice, she, for her part, would leave them free to live their own lives.

At the McLarens' Rukhmabai was primarily engaged in preparing for the preliminary examination which she needed to pass to qualify for admission to the School of Medicine. Her biggest dread at the time was whether she would be able to pass this examination. Her state of mind at that time is described in the London-based *Indian Female Evangelist*. Reporting that Rukhmabai was 'much perplexed as to what her course shall be', the paper wrote: 'She came over to this country, in the hope that she might qualify as a lady doctor, and devote herself to the relief of her country women, but she finds the study of Medicine extremely difficult and is much disheartened. We ought to remember her in our prayers.'[9] The pessimism is echoed in another assessment of Rukhmabai: 'There is talk of making her a doctor and sending her back to India, but it seems at present doubtful whether she has the strength and nerve for the ordeal of a medical training.' This, it may be noted, was the assessment of one who thought highly of Rukhmabai:

> She seems in the solitude of her upbringing to have thought out and solved for herself on the most advanced lines nearly all social problems of the day. Her friends here find that they have nothing to teach her; and she sometimes nearly blows the roofs of their heads off by the daring doctrines which she announces.[10]

Cornelia Sorabji, too, did not expect Rukhmabai to pass the qualifying examination.[11]

Incidentally, all the three assessments were based on conversations with Rukhmabai. She would all her life remain the honest, guileless person these conversations reflect.

Be that as it may, she chose to take the Society of Apothecaries of London Examination in Arts. The examination consisted of five subjects: Botany, Euclid, Algebra, Arithmetic and English. She had more than a year to pass this examination, for the plan was for her to commence her medical studies from the academic year beginning October 1890. She decided to spread out her preparation for the preliminary examination and clear it in two instalments. She gave herself eleven months before taking, in March 1890, the examination in Botany and Euclid. She cleared the remaining three subjects in June.

A big load was off her chest. She had averted the disgrace of failing to follow the coveted course. Her own intelligence and application apart, the result was in no small measure due to the gentle guidance of her hosts and the concentrated studies that staying with them permitted.

Even while Rukhmabai was occupied with the qualifying examination, she and Eva found ample time to talk about their common passion, women's cause. Eva was by this time in the forefront of the rapidly burgeoning suffragist movement. The moving spirit behind the Women's Liberal Association of Crewe – her husband's parliamentary constituency – she was also an active member of the Women's Liberal Federation. The Women's Liberal Association of Crewe was part of a wide network of similar local associations which women had formed under the aegis of the Liberal Party. The Women's Liberal Federation was set up, two years before Rukhmabai's arrival, to coordinate the activities of the various Women's Liberal

Associations. An indefatigable crusader, Eva also wrote extensively. All her feminist efforts were fully supported by her husband.

Eva McLaren's relationship with Rukhmabai was not soiled by the condescension that usually marks benefactor-beneficiary interactions. As a result, Rukhmabai learnt much from that fortunate association. Eva rid Rukhmabai of some of her naivety and made available a larger perspective for understanding things. For example, Rukhmabai had seen through the Indian male reformers' protestations for women's welfare and, consequently, insisted on legislation by the British Indian rulers. She innocently assumed that the British would readily agree to legislate.

The same innocence led her to appeal on behalf of her Indian sisters to Victoria, the Queen-Empress:

> This 50th year of our Queen's accession to the most renowned throne is the jubilee year in which every town and every village in her dominions is to show their loyalty in the best way it can and wish the Mother-Queen a long happy life to rule over us for many years with peace and prosperity. At such an unusual occasion will the mother listen to an earnest appeal from her millions of Indian daughters for a few simple words of change into the books of Hindoo law – that 'marriages performed before the respective ages of 20 in boys and 15 in girls shall not be considered legal in the eyes of law if brought before the Court.'[12]

Believing, as did most educated Indians of the day, in the civilizing mission of the British, Rukhmabai assumed that women in Britain were an enviable community. Early during her stay in London, she said: 'If we only had one-eighth of what you women of England have, we should be content.'[13]

She needed to learn that the depravity she had recognized was not peculiar to Indian males. That learning, ironically, came from being among the same British women whose lot she had envied. And it began under the protective care of Eva McLaren who had sensed the naivety that lurked behind young Rukhmabai's courage, conviction and intelligence. Eva also realized that she had to operate delicately, in full recognition of Rukhmbai's exceptionality and without aggravating her brittle self-esteem.

Eva set about informing Rukhmabai about British public life in general and about the British women's movement in particular. True to her concern for the poor since her early social work days, Eva took care to draw Rukhmabai's attention to the condition and problems of the working classes as well. In fact, the very first act of public concern that Eva encouraged Rukhmabai to perform within weeks of her arrival was to donate two and a half shillings to the Alverthorpe Weavers' Fund. Eva herself made a similar donation. The Fund was meant to provide relief to the 130-odd female weavers of a mill in Alverthorpe who had gone on a strike against a drastic reduction in their wages.

Eva also began, simultaneously, to bring Rukhmabai gradually into the women's movement. As a first step, at two meetings of women in the neighbouring towns of Crewe and Sandbach, Eva spoke on the condition of women in India and described at length the struggle waged by Rukhmabai. This led to Rukhmabai being invited to speak, the following month, at those women's Conversazione in the Town Hall of Crewe.

Before the year 1889 ended, Eva arranged for Rukhmabai to travel to Edinburgh and participate in the annual meeting of the Edinburgh National Society for Women's Suffrage. Here, following her plan to slowly shake Rukhmabai out of her dread of public speaking, Eva persuaded her to make a small intervention by seconding a motion that called for parliamentary suffrage for women.

The plan was a spectacular success. Within a year, on 10 July 1890, Rukhmabai was making her maiden public speech before a large audience inside Bristol's Tyndale Chapel. She, the local press reported, 'spoke in the refined tone of an educated lady'.[14] Her speech, which dealt with the condition of women in India, was followed, fittingly enough, by a collection for the Indian Zenana Mission.[15]

From her hesitant appearance at the Conversazione in Crewe to her impressive solo performance in Bristol, the Hindu Lady had come a long way in just one year. Her gradual induction in public life and the women's movement was complete. Preparations to enter the medical school had not prevented her association with the movement. Nor would regular medical studies.

A little digression may be in order here. The invitations that started pouring in gave Rukhmabai a chance to see different parts of the country and experience the United Kingdom's socio-cultural-political heterogeneity. Take, for instance, her visit to Edinburgh. Apart from being mesmerized by the city's magical beauty, she learnt a critical lesson: Scotland was significantly different from England. England was not Britain.

Moreover, in Edinburgh, where she had come along with the McLarens, Rukhmabai stayed with Walter's mother, Priscilla Bright McLaren, the president of the Edinburgh National Society for Women's Suffrage. Besides being someone in her own right, Priscilla, we may recall, was sister of John Bright and her late husband, Duncan, had been an influential MP. Rukhmabai saw the power and influence the women of the family exercised as much in Edinburgh as in London.

Welcomed among the elite of British society, she ruefully thought of the regular meetings of the best minds of the day at her stepfather's residence. Had the social arrangements been different in India, she would have learnt so much from those minds. Let alone the outsiders, even her stepfather's fine mind was beyond access.

To return to where we digressed, the coming together of Rukhmabai and the 'women's rights' women' was the coming together of fellow sufferers. Rukhmabai was buoyed up by those fellow sufferers' determination to fight their own fights.

The British women's movement gave her a larger and chastening perspective. She had nurtured a flattering image of women in Britain; that is what had prompted her, from distant Bombay, to ask them to support their suffering Indian sisters. Now that she was in Britain, she could see that British women were themselves engaged in a hard struggle to claim their basic rights and dignity vis-à-vis men. Ironically, they were engaged in that hard struggle as subjects of the same Queen to whom she had appealed for the gift of a 'mere sentence' on behalf of her Indian daughters.

Partially disabused of her innocence, Rukhmabai could see that, not only the male social reformers she had seen back home, but men in general would not act unless women acted on their own behalf. She also saw that nearly all the local Women's Liberal Associations, as also their umbrella organization, the Women's Liberal Federation, owed their formation to the lead taken by dedicated individual women.

Rukhmabai realized that similar efforts were needed in India, and thought she must make the vital first move. Within months of reaching London, she was bubbling with plans to form a Ladies' Association for Indian women. So irresistible was her enthusiasm that in her first meeting with the freshly arrived Cornelia Sorabji, of whom she knew precious little, Rukhmabai excitedly laid out the scheme before her. She was keen to enlist this bright Parsi to the cause.

Cornelia was not enthused. Reporting their conversation to her family the following day, she wrote: 'She [Rukhmabai] is bent on some grand scheme for a Ladies Association for which she wishes to raise funds.' 'I wish,' Cornelia continued, 'all Indian women would work steadily and usefully instead of aiming at original schemes. I feel that about myself. There are too many unfinished projects extant in India.' She concluded caustically: 'I told Rukhmabai she ought to help Ramabai, but that would be second fiddle.'[16]

Four months later, reporting to her parents an interview Rukhmabai had with Lord Harris, the Under-Secretary of State for India, Cornelia wrote: '... and she most amusingly appeared as the champion of Female Education in India! Did you ever? ... I suggested that a visit here brought responsibilities, and that we ought to seek usefulness not notoriety and fame. She is quite spoilt and thinks no end of herself.'[17]

Rukhmabai felt frustrated. If promising young Indian women like Cornelia were to be indifferent, indeed hostile, to the cause of their sisters, the scheme would be harder to implement than she had thought. But, animated by the spirit of the British women's movement and encouragement from the likes of the McLarens and Millicent Anderson Fawcett, she persisted with the scheme for a while.

The British, both women and men, looked up to Rukhmabai as an exemplar, and the British feminists were glad to have her in their midst. This, however, did not affect their presumption that, no matter what their societal failings, the British were superior to Indians. Imperial instincts were not a male monopoly. The white man's burden was also the white woman's burden.

Rukhmabai, for the British, was not only an exemplar but also an example: an example of what the British civilizing mission had achieved in India. Rukhmabai herself accepted the secular superiority of the British. Following the epistemic hold the British exercised over them, many Indians had accepted their rulers' civilizing mission. There was also, moreover, the empirical contrast that whereas middle-class British women were fighting for better education, employment and suffrage, those in India were not getting even primary education.

There was also a Christian evangelical angle to the celebration of Rukhmabai in Britain. This is best revealed in the following description of what preceded Rukhmabai's lecture at the Tyndale Chapel:

> After singing and prayer Mr Fry [the chairman] spoke of the responsibility placed upon us in relation to our people in India. The country has not been given for our own aggrandisement. If we are to govern India, we must be very particular about the laws we enact, and the English Government should not uphold any customs which involve suffering for the women of India. If England is to hold her right positions among the nations, she must govern those who are brought under her sway righteously. Nothing short of the blessed Gospel of Jesus Christ can purify and sanctify the people of that land.[18]

But Rukhmabai cared little for Christianity. At the time of leaving India, she did not have a moment's hesitation in assuring her anxious mother that she would not accept Christianity. That assurance had sprung from faith. That faith was never shaken.

To return to what had brought her to London, Rukhmabai continued to be apprehensive even after clearing the qualifying examination. This brought no assurance that she had it in her to comprehend the totally unfamiliar technical subjects that would make her a doctor. In terms of her educational inadequacy, though, Rukhmabai was no worse off than most of her British counterparts. Like in India, very few girls in nineteenth-century Britain received formal schooling. They studied at home, with a tutor, and only a few went to one of the colleges (in London and a few elsewhere) that provided schooling to girls. Rukhmabai herself had joined the Queen's College to prepare for the pre-medical examination.

Yet, she was more disadvantaged than were the British female students. Unlike them, she had to do the course in a language which was not her own and in which she had received no formal teaching prior to coming to England. The compulsion to study those esoteric subjects and, worse, to be tested in them in a language she was not proficient in, was a virtual nightmare.

The nightmare, fortunately, did not last long. Two favourable circumstances saved Rukhmabai. The first was the warmth and intimacy that characterized the London School of Medicine for Women. When Rukhmabai joined it, the School was still instinct with the missionary spirit that had brought it into being fifteen years ago. Hailed as the 'Mother school of all medical women in Great Britain and Ireland', it had, with its 100-plus students in the year Rukhmabai joined it, retained its character as a harmonic extended family and not grown into an impersonal professional educational institution. Founded to wipe out the disgrace of women's inferiority and inequality, the School was committed to sending out women doctors who would carry forward their alma mater's mission and facilitate women's medical education.

All these factors made for a pattern of teaching and interaction between teachers and students that extended beyond the class-room. The teachers, especially the three female teachers – the others were men – followed each student's performance, attended to her particular problems and kept her motivated. There was also the founding secretary of the School, Miss Heaton, who mothered the students like her own. Whatever their need, she was there to turn to.

Viewing their students as potential missionaries, the School personnel felt a personal stake in the shaping and success of each student. They felt it a little more keenly in Rukhmabai's case. She was a co-fighter in the cause of women. She had come to the School to train to serve her unhappy sisters. It also mattered that Rukhmabai was sent by one of the founders of the School, Dr Pechey, and her application for admission recommended by a never-failing friend of the School, Elizabeth Manning. Furthermore, Millicent Garrett

Fawcett, one of the leading lights of the British women's movement and younger sister of the School's Dean, Dr Garrett Anderson, greatly admired Rukhmabai and had written about her in the November 1890 issue of the *Contemporary Review*. And Dr Mary Scharlieb, who taught Midwifery at the School, had earlier served in India and become particularly concerned about Indian women.

Even before Rukhmabai joined the School, her teachers knew that their prize student would need special care and guidance. Solicitous though they were about all their students, there was more at stake in the success of this student. Her success would be a matter of special pride – and a great advertisement – for the School. Thus, in the School's official report for 1890–91, Rukhmabai's first year, she was described as one of its most promising students. Later, when Isabel Thorne, the School's Honorary Secretary who was also one of its founders and a member of the 'Edinburgh Seven', wrote for promotional publication a survey of the first thirty years of the School, she thought it worthwhile to include the following:

> In 1890 Rukhmabai was amongst the new students. She is a Hindu lady whose refusal to carry out a marriage made for her in childhood caused considerable agitation on the question in Bombay. After a successful student career she qualified and returned to India, where she continues to do excellent work.[19]

These teachers put in that extra bit for Rukhmabai and induced in her the belief that she had it in her to be a good doctor.

Rukhmabai was also helped by her own gradual realization that she knew better English than she believed. How the complex about her poor English paralyzed her is illustrated by an event that occurred when she had already been in London for six months. She was at a lecture by Cornelia Sorabji on women in India. After the lecture was over, the organizers wanted her also to comment. Their request froze her. 'She could not be prevailed on to speak, as she did not yet feel herself sufficiently fluent in our language.'[20]

Rukhmabai's complex is also revealed in the way she irritated Cornelia Sorabji by her persistent protestations of being deficient in English in sharp contrast to Cornelia. As against these protestations, Cornelia wrote about Rukhmabai: 'She speaks English ever so much better now.'[21] It was three months after this attestation that Rukhmabai was petrified by the request to speak after Cornelia's lecture. In fact, as early as March 1887 when Rukhmabai was still in Bombay, a missionary Englishwoman had written:

> It was a delight to hear her speak English, her use of it was so pure and just fluent enough to be pretty. It was bookish English, but on her lips the long, unconversational words sounded quaint and charming. She said she had learned to speak our language from an English lady who came in often to talk with her, and she added, 'It has been a great help to me to read the English authors. I am now reading Goldsmith, and find him very interesting.'[22]

Self-perception, not incompetence, had crippled Rukhmabai.

She started learning English late and for quite a while was not able to think in it. She would first formulate in Marathi what she wanted to say, mentally translate it into English and then speak it out. That made her delivery in English slow and halting, and she would feel awkward while speaking the language. The awkwardness was aggravated by the awareness that the English she spoke was bookish, quaint and unconversational.

To speak English was a strain for Rukhmabai. The strain was comparatively less in interpersonal conversation. While the other person spoke, she would have time to think of her response and translate it in her mind. That was not possible while speaking in public, unless she had prepared beforehand. We may never know when Rukhmabai began speaking English effortlessly, unvexed by the need for pre-verbal translation. But things seem to have fallen into place in time to make pleasant her four years at the medical school.

One of the nicer things that happened was her admission to London's prestigious College Hall. She was lucky that her sponsors, unlike the general run of donors, did not worry about their pennies and sent her to this delightful abode. The Hall had been started in 1882 by a group of feminists including Eva McLaren's sister, Henrietta Muller, to provide a collegiate residence for women studying at the University College or the London School of Medicine for Women. Accommodating thirty-six residents, its building included a large dining hall, a drawing room, and smaller rooms in which the residents could entertain their friends. There was also a library stocked with books relating to the resident students' courses. The Hall was just a leisurely eight-minute walk – 700 yards – from the School.

The College Hall, with its small number of residents and cosmopolitan composition, conduced to a camaraderie that helped Rukhmabai get over the wrench of leaving the McLaren home. It also facilitated the formation of some very warm friendships. One of those was with Aldrich Blake, one year Rukhmabai's senior at the LSMW, the future Dame Louisa who would make a name as Britain's first female surgeon. Aldrich was the one who would help Rukhmabai choose the equipment for her medical work in India.

The bedrooms in the Hall were provided with every comfort. However, the residents were free to furnish and decorate their rooms the way they liked. As they came from different parts of the world, the rooms presented a variety of tastes, including ostentation. Rukhmabai's room was marked by a combination of austerity and elegance. That elegant austerity, in fact, was the defining, and most endearing, feature of her being. It was reflected in her speech, her writing, her dress, indeed her entire demeanour.

And there was the quiet grace of her beauty. From Chief Justice

Sargent inside the courtroom and the missionary Englishwoman in Bombay to the countless who saw her in Britain, there was no one who missed it.

She was never ostentatious. Not even on festive or ceremonial occasions. Here is a description of her at the School's inaugural lecture for 1891. Rukhmabai, so goes the description, was 'very quietly dressed … in a loose grey robe, a sort of compromise between the native and English dress'. The full import of this description comes out as we read on and meet the wife of a doctor from Bengal – one Mrs Roy – who was present on the occasion. In stark contrast to Rukhmabai, and typically for Indians in Britain, Mrs Roy was 'a dazzling object, attired in the most gorgeous of Oriental costumes and splendid jewels'.[23]

This was only the second year of Rukhmabai as a student in a foreign land, and already she had no use for extraneous props to make a mark. Self-assured and happy to be left alone, she was untroubled by the pressure to impress others.

Even in the primarily external matter of dress, she followed her aesthetic instincts instead of choosing from the available readymade options. Displaying a talent for sartorial innovation that has remained unrecognized, she designed something subdued and pleasing that not only accorded with her temperament and lifestyle, but was also eminently functional. Indeed, its functionality deserves special mention. After Dr Anandibai Joshee's premature death on account of her strict observance, in the cold of Philadelphia, of the Hindu sartorial norms of a temperate climate, Indians, especially women, going to the West had become very anxious about protecting themselves. Cornelia Sorabji put it rather bluntly when, explaining why she 'submitted' to flannel clothes, she wrote: 'I do not want to be a second Anandibai Joshi.'[24] Rukhmabai for her part had the imagination to design an agreeable 'compromise between the native and English dress.'

Rukhmabai applied for admission to the London School of Medicine for Women on 29 September 1890. Two days later, on 1 October, she was listening to the inaugural lecture with which, traditionally, began the School's academic year. A special feature of the School's calendar, the lecture, as distinct from the specialized information they would get in their classes, was meant to educate the students in larger issues of the practice, problems and philosophy of medicine.

The inaugural lecture was a tradition followed by most of Britain's medical schools. However, the visionary founders of the School of Medicine for Women used the tradition to promote their institution's primary objective. They had followed an unwritten rule that, exceptions apart, only women who had made a mark in their chosen fields would be invited. Even among the women lecturers, preference was given to those who had distinguished themselves in the field of medicine. Since this was the first school in the country that provided medical education to women, it was only natural that the majority of speakers came from among the School's promoters and alumni. As it happened, all the inaugural lectures organized during Rukhmabai's studentship were delivered by old students of the School.

A striking feature of the inaugural lecture was that the first row was reserved for the first-year students, not for the distinguished invitees.

The lecture for 1890 was delivered by Dr Florence Nightingale Boyd, MD. Also present on the occasion, as a special invitee and speaker, was Elizabeth Blackwell. One of the founders of the School, Dr Blackwell was a venerable mother figure who, by her example, had inspired her countrywomen to dream of being doctors. Elizabeth was already twenty-six when, moved by a long ailing female friend's lament that she would not have suffered like she did if she had had a woman doctor, she resolved to become one. Of the several institutions she applied to, only one – the Geneva Medical College, supported by its male students' vote – admitted her.

That was in New York. It was another Elizabeth who, following Blackwell's example, became the first woman to qualify as a doctor in Britain. This was Elizabeth Garrett Anderson, the Dean of the London School of Medicine for Women. Backed by her rich businessman father, she applied to various medical schools in Britain and was denied admission by all. She thereupon decided to stoop to conquer. She became a nurse.

Behind her stooping is an inspirational story. Elizabeth's father had brought her to London to meet the city's leading doctors and seek their help. What she got was polite indifference at best and undisguised hostility at worst. There was, though, one well-meaning physician who, suggesting an 'appropriate' option, asked Elizabeth:

'My dear lady, why not become a nurse?'

'Because I prefer to earn a thousand, rather than twenty pounds a year,' riposted young Elizabeth.[25]

The same plucky Elizabeth pocketed her pride and became a nurse. As a nurse, she employed all her intelligence, perseverance and tact to win over one teacher after another and gained their permission to attend their classes. At times she also had to take private lectures from recognized teachers and pay them ten times the money that she paid for regular classes. Finally, she used a certain loophole in the existing rules to take the examination of the Society of Apothecaries and became a doctor virtually on the sly. What followed is described in Sophia Jex-Blake's *Medical Women*:

But no sooner had she thus demonstrated the existence of at least a postern gate by which women might enter the profession, than the authorities took alarm, and, with the express object of preventing other women from following so terrible a precedent, a rule was passed, forbidding students henceforth to receive any part of their education privately, it being well known that women would be rigorously excluded from some at least of the public classes![26]

This book had made a profound impact on Rukhmabai. And here, four years later, she was in the presence of the two pathbreaking Elizabeths. Even as, settled in the front row, she nervously looked forward to an abstruse exposition, there followed a most solicitous discourse on the freshers' problems and ways to overcome them.

Boyd began by telling the teachers that what the students needed the least was to be told to work well. Rather, they needed to be warned against overstudy. Overstudy ruined their health and made them indifferent to the claims and interests of others. She exhorted the students to be relaxed, take care of their health and remember that a small body like the students of the School must stand united and consider the good of the community as their own.

Finally, she advised the students to be sensitive to the state of society and avoid extreme views and conduct. Those who had done the most to better the social condition of women had proved that they could take up an independent course and yet remain women to the core. This was Boyd's counter to the prevailing belief that becoming doctors robbed women of their womanly qualities. Of that the two trailblazing Elizabeths were living evidence.

Boyd's lecture rid Rukhmabai of many a demon. So did Elizabeth Garrett Anderson's motherly advice on the occasion. She, the School's dean, told the students to be as much in the open air as possible, eat three good meals a day and drink various teas.

Useful though Boyd's inaugural lecture was, it was the one Dr Mary Emily Dowson gave the following year that opened a new horizon for Rukhmabai and the other students. A brilliant former student of the School, Dowson had become the first qualified female surgeon in Britain and Ireland. Hers was a plea for a holistic approach. She called upon the students to acquire general knowledge and culture, and not be content with mere technical information. It was necessary, Dowson maintained, to know something of everything to know much of something. General knowledge and culture provided safeguards against fads and professional bigotry, and saved doctors from becoming mindless diagnostic machines.

A patient, Dowson emphasized, was not a patchwork of bodily signs and symptoms made after a common pattern. Every patient was a unique, reasoning human being with a psychical as well as physiological aspect. As a unique being, the patient would require from the physician more than mere acquaintance with physiology. The physician had to guard against being over-instructed and under-educated.

Leaving the students in no doubt that her critique was aimed at the male mafia of diagnostic machines that would not let women enter the medical profession and humanize it, Dowson concluded with the exhortation that no female doctor should become 'a female copy of the practical man'.[27] Listening to this stirring, brilliant lecture, Rukhmabai must have felt vindicated afresh. She had in her 'Letters of a Hindu Lady' done what Dowson was doing that day: lay bare the scheming of males and their collective blindness to what they did.

Marking a break from convention, there was no inaugural lecture in 1892. Instead, an informal meeting of the students and friends of the School was organized on the opening day. This had a special attraction for Rukhmabai because Pechey Phipson was among the invited guests.

The last inaugural lecture during Rukhmabai's years at the School was delivered by Dr Helen Webb on 2 October 1893. Like Dowson in 1891, Webb, too, advised the students to take a broad view of the work before them. In medicine, she emphasized, there is no such thing as an isolated fact. The systems of the human body must be studied separately, but they cannot be known without grasping their mutual relations in the body as a whole. Each step in the great art of healing is but part of a great whole, and each step must be followed by its own consequences. A good doctor must learn to combine a reverence for accuracy of detail with an understanding of the interrelationships of things.

Further, articulating the philosophy of the London School of Medicine for Women, Webb exhorted the students to combine the best of womanhood with the highest proficiency in medicine. Highest technical proficiency would make them, as physicians and surgeons, the equal of their male counterparts. The best of womanhood would distinguish them from their male counterparts in that they would be doctors with an awakened social conscience: dignified, reflective and well-rounded professionals for whom individual well-being was inseparable from collective well-being. Their being such doctors would belie the belief that women were unfit for the medical profession.

Rukhmabai was most struck by Webb's formulation that 'the highest ideal of the medical profession (perhaps never to be realized)' was to work towards 'a state of things in which its own existence will no longer be called for.' Implicit in this ideal was a radical shift from the cure of disease to its prevention. As Webb put it:

> In the good old times, when a fever or plague broke out its presence became at once an accepted fact, and professional energy was altogether directed to the cure of cases as they emerged. It is most significant of the times that during the present outbreak of cholera in Europe the literature of the subject has almost altogether dealt with discovery of the sources of infection and their speedy destruction.[28]

This marked the beginning of Rukhmabai's interest in the emerging field of preventive medicine, which she studied before returning to India.

Rukhmabai was seriously concerned with the question of what it meant to practise medicine. To educate herself better and broaden her horizon, she began attending public lectures by eminent doctors, especially those by her favourite women of medicine: Elizabeth Blackwell, Elizabeth Garrett Anderson and Mary Scharlieb.

Suffering had induced Rukhmabai early in life to go to the roots of things and inclined her towards a life of service. The inaugural lectures furnished her with an inspirational perspective to reflect on the *raison d'etre* of the medical profession. By the time she left the School, she had internalized its vision of 'female professionalism'. Aspiring to supplant the reigning male professionalism, female professionalism was marked by social maternalism, public conscience and concern for the local community. This would make her a selfless, caring doctor and a person at peace with herself.

To turn from foundational issues to the details of School life, Rukhmabai was lucky that the year she joined, the School building in Handel Street had been enlarged and suitably modified. Its 100-plus students now had excellent classrooms, a fine chemical laboratory and an anatomy room as good as any in Britain. The entire class teaching was conducted here. For practical work the students walked across the short pleasant path leading to the Royal Free Hospital in Euston road for bedside and clinical instruction, training in patient care, and as clerks and dressers.

The Hospital's operating room was the venue for practical training in all kinds of surgery. Surgery was a subject of special concern for the School authorities. Women those days were believed to be physically and physiologically unfit for surgery. Here is a telling example. Rukhmabai had just joined the School, when Elizabeth Garrett Anderson testified before a House of Lords Committee. When she told the Committee that the New Hospital – staffed entirely by women and catering only to women and children – provided even surgical facilities, a member asked her in barely concealed disbelief: 'Do you think that women have strength enough of wrist to do those things?' Garrett Anderson simply answered, 'Yes.' But, then, towards the very end when she thought the Committee was done with her, another member shot forth: 'Would your experience lead you to think that it takes your lady students longer to get used to the terrible sights and scenes in the operating theatre than it would men students?' Clearly, Garrett Anderson's earlier cryptic 'Yes' had failed to shake the Committee's conviction that women were naturally ill-equipped to be doctors. This time she told them with unconcealed sarcasm:

> I have had very little experience of men students. I do not know if I have ever heard of any of our women fainting; I have heard of men fainting occasionally; but I daresay it takes both of them a little time to get used to it. I have never known of a woman leaving off the study of medicine because she found it too dreadful. They soon become deeply interested in it.[29]

So long as this prejudice prevailed, female doctors would not command the respect that the School was founded to get them. It could not do that without sending out alumni who were second to no male surgeon in their adroitness with the scalpel. That required excellent training in surgery for the students. This was not happening.

There were practical difficulties. The Royal Free Hospital's operating room, where the School sent its students for training, could accommodate around twenty students. But it was so badly arranged that, except for those in the front, most others could see very little or nothing. Over this the School authorities had little control. However, they were scrupulous in following the regulations of the medical council and designing their teaching exactly on the lines of the men's medical schools.

Rukhmabai was a dedicated and hard-working student. But she found the going tough for a while. Except in one subject, her marks during the first two years were not promising. In Anatomy, she got 48 out of 100 marks, as against the highest of 82 and the lowest of 22. She stood literally in the middle with nine students above and nine below her. In Physiology, she got 33 as against the highest of 90 and the lowest of five, with 18 students above and seven below her. In Medicine, she got 45 out of 100 as against the highest of 89 and lowest of 37, with 23 students above and only two below her. In Midwifery, a high-scoring subject, she got 70 out of 100, as against the highest of 98 and lowest of 15, with 28 students above and 20 below her. In Gynaecology, another high-scoring subject, she got only 45, as against the highest of 98 and lowest of 20, with 40 students above and only eight below her. In Operative Midwifery, with 100 out of 150 marks, she stood again in the middle, with eight students above and eight below her. In Surgery, which carried a maximum of 400 marks, Rukhmabai, along with six other students, failed to submit her papers in time.

This level of performance would not make her a doctor. But she was not unduly worried. She believed she was an abler student than her marks indicated. Besides, she was determined to succeed. Her stakes were enormous. Failure would shatter all her dreams; and it would cause her the humiliation of letting down the many well-wishers who, reposing faith in her, had generously supported her.

She had only two years to improve her performance. To pass the Triple Qualification examination that she had chosen to sit, she would need to score at least 55 per cent marks in every paper. In the event, she not only passed, but did so in her first attempt. No less creditably, she passed it immediately upon the completion of the prescribed minimum of forty-five months of formal study and training. Very few students managed to pass so fast and in their first attempt.

Seen against her indifferent initial academic record, this achievement speaks of Rukhmabai's ability, application and will. It speaks also of her personal ethics. Grateful to her benefactors, she was loath to burden them with a farthing more than was absolutely necessary. On 1 October 1890 commenced her medical studies. On 30 June 1894 was completed the mandatory forty-five-month period of her studies. On 5 July, post-haste, she had applied for the Triple Qualification examination in Edinburgh.

Commendable as the achievement was, there is another side to it. In travelling to distant Edinburgh to sit the Triple Qualification examination, Rukhmabai had purposely avoided the more prestigious examination of the London University. Besides being more expensive, compared to the Triple Qualification, this was also a very difficult examination. Rukhmabai's School authorities themselves encouraged only their best students to sit the London examination. They knew that every student of theirs who passed this examination would bring the School extra credit; but they also needed to avoid the adverse publicity that would accrue from the failure of their students.

That she cleared the Triple Qualification in her first attempt and prudently avoided the London University examination, these two facts together offer a realistic appraisal of Rukhmabai's mettle as a student. However, the fact that to avoid the London examination she was obliged to go all the way to Edinburgh hides yet another gender inequity to which women aspiring to be doctors were subjected in the UK. Unlike the relatively mediocre students of the London School of Medicine for Women, male students of similar academic calibre did not have to travel to distant unknown cities. Easier options abounded for them in or around wherever they were studying.

Following Elizabeth Garrett's cunning exploitation of the then existing rules to become a doctor, the medical profession had slammed its doors shut in the face of future female aspirants. It was a whole decade later, in 1877, that the King's and Queen's College of Physicians in Dublin and soon thereafter the University of London initiated a gingerly process of opening the medical profession to women. Then, in 1884, the Royal Colleges of Physicians and Surgeons of Edinburgh and the Faculty of Physicians and Surgeons of Glasgow jointly instituted their 'Triple Qualification' examination and admitted to it female candidates equally with male candidates. These three were the only examinations open to women in the entire United Kingdom of Great Britain and Ireland.

In fairness to Rukhmabai, it may be added that while Triple Qualifications offered a relatively easier option, it was by no means an easy examination. The compulsory courses that the examinees had to clear were very comprehensive. Numbering thirteen, these were: Anatomy, Practical Anatomy, Pathological Anatomy, Physiology, Chemistry, Practical or Analytical Chemistry, Materia Medica, Practice of Medicine, Clinical Medicine, Practice and Principles of Surgery, Clinical Surgery, Midwifery and Diseases of Women and Children, and Medical Jurisprudence. In addition, the prospective examinees were strongly advised to get instructed in certain allied courses, such as Gynaecology, Ophthalmic, Aural and Mental Diseases, Natural History and Comparative Anatomy, the use of the microscope and its application to medicine and physiology, and at least three months' study of fevers under recognized clinical instructors. Finally, the examinees were also required to possess certificates of having attended at least six cases of labour; twenty-four months of medical and surgical practice in a general hospital; six months (or three months with three months' hospital clerkship) of practice in a recognized public dispensary; three months' instruction in practical pharmacy; instruction in the theory and practice of vaccination; and six weeks of operations performed under the teacher's supervision.

No less important in this context is the fact that Rukhmabai had done nineteen courses, six more than the thirteen prescribed for Triple Qualification. These included Preventive Medicine, Dentistry and the emerging specialities of Mental Pathology and Ophthalmic Surgery. She did this to maximize her competence as a physician and surgeon. She also sought for her training in specific subjects hospitals known for their specialized excellence. Thus, after completing her studies at the School, she briefly studied at the Leeds School of Medicine before returning to London where she gained further experience at the Royal Free Hospital. She went all the way to Dublin to acquire practical experience at the city's famous maternity hospital, the Rotunda. Rukhmabai also trained for three months in practical dentistry at the National Dental Hospital. Knowing that her work would be among women and children, she also served for a while at a children's hospital.

After clearing the Triple Qualification, Rukhmabai also obtained the MD of the University of Brussels.

Clearing Triple Qualification apart, her visit to Edinburgh this time became memorable for Rukhmabai for another noteworthy reason. She stayed with the legendary Sophia Jex-Blake. In her *Life of Dr Sophia Jex-Blake*, Dr Margaret Todd writes: 'When Rukhmabai came to Edinburgh for her Final Professional Examination, she was S.J.-B.'s guest, and a strong mutual admiration and friendship was the result.'[30] In fact, not only the great S.J.-B. but even her dear friend and biographer, Margaret Todd, became fond of Rukhmabai.

For her part, Rukhmabai had worshipped S.J.-B. since she read her *Medical Women*. S.J.-B., too, had admired Rukhmabai since then through letters from Pechey and the celebratory coverage of her case in the British press. Each saw the other as a crusader. That mutual admiration flowered into friendship during Rukhmabai's stay at S.J.-B's charming Bruntsfield Lodge.

Luckily this happened when Rukhmabai had come for the Triple Qualifications examination. Just being with S.J.-B. charged her with an energy she had not known before. That and precious tips from the charismatic hostess helped Rukhmabai surpass herself.

She also learnt something about a different kind of life. S.J.-B. lived with Margaret Todd who was nineteen years her junior and about the same age as Rukhmabai. Beginning as S.J.-B.'s student, Margaret became a friend and partner. Margaret's book on S.J.-B., written after the latter's death, was an act of love, loyalty and remembrance. They lived together honestly and discreetly, neither flaunting nor denying their intimacy. It is a pity that we do not know what, with her post-London conservatism, Rukhmabai thought of that beautiful, tender relationship.

One of her best and lasting friendships in London was struck with Alys Pearsall Smith. The same age as Rukhmabai, Alys was the daughter of an American Quaker couple who were friends with the McLarens. It is a measure of their friendship that when, a little before returning to India, Rukhmabai issued an appeal for funds for a girls' school in Bombay, Alys was one of the two women to whom the subscribers were asked to send money. Also, Alys' mother, Hannah Whitall Smith, was so impressed with Rukhmabai that she wrote a long article, entitled 'A Hindu Heroine: A Sketch of Rukhmabai', which appeared in the *Woman's Signal* of 25 October 1894.

While this friendship was forming, Alys fell in love with a young aristocrat who would soon burst into fame in the world of philosophy and into notoriety in British public life as a dissenter. This was Bertrand Russell. Being privy to the unfolding of this rocky romance was for Rukhmabai an altogether new and exciting experience. She saw that even in a society where the young enjoyed considerable freedom of choice, family pressure could make life difficult for them. Russell's grandmother – a domineering aristocrat whose husband was twice prime minister of Great Britain – left no stone unturned to prevent her beloved 'Bertie's' union with a commoner from the United States.

Notwithstanding the hiccups in her American friend's romance, Rukhmabai could not miss the contrast between India and Britain. She thought of her widowed childhood friend, Shanta, who would not remarry despite her erudite father's impassioned entreaties. And here was Alys – a puritan and not a free thinker like Russell – who felt drawn to a man and managed to get married to him. Rukhmabai was also struck by the easy acceptance of her friend's affair even though she was five years older than her lover. In India, where old men routinely married pre-pubescent virgins, this would have caused a scandal.

If Mohini Varde is to be trusted, Rukhmabai harboured a lifelong aversion to love and marriage. Obviously reproducing the family legend, Varde writes:

> She could not accept the friendships between men and women. Though she was friendly with all the girls in her hostel, she expressed her displeasure when one of the inmates went out with a male doctor. Rakhmabai's mind definitely bore impressions of the past, for one cannot come across any further instances in her life where she related intimately with any member of the opposite sex.[31]

Produced by her traumatic past, this antipathy, according to Varde, was reinforced by the lifelong hold that Victorian morality had on Rukhmabai.

Fortunately, Rukhmabai's youth was not altogether so desolate and deprived. She struck in London a lively friendship with a member of the opposite sex. The account of that friendship, unfortunately, comes from Cornelia Sorabji. She wrote on 2 February 1890:

> She has taken a great fancy to a stuck-up fop from Kolapoor, the most despicable youth I've ever set eyes on – who is reading for the C.S. and spent a Vac in France, with the result that he dresses and talks [like a] 'masher' [a man who makes passes at women] now and wears his hair in furbellows [sic] around his head. I loathed him the first time I saw him, when at Miss Manning's he talked big about his attainments and expressed his indignation at being taken

for an Abyssinian Prince – 'that black fellow'. – as he said with the worst taste possible, seeing his complexion and his remarks were present at the same time. His name is Mutgatkar. And Miss Mailey told me that he and Rukhmabai wander about the streets together – most disgraceful I call it. That comes of opposing existing laws, and breaking loose from proper restraint.[32]

Cornelia's visceral dislike for Rukhmabai runs through her too-lurid-to-be-credible narrative. Read against the grain, it provides a tantalizing glimpse of a joyous interlude in young Rukhmabai's lonely, sad life. It was a most unlikely – and therefore wonderful – interlude. It was happening, we may recall, to the woman who, not long back, had dismissed that romantic bestseller, *A Roman Singer*, for containing 'nothing but mere love matters'. She, in the prime of her youth, had been condemned by law and custom to remain single all her life. Even while eschewing all pleasures, she had been publicly portrayed as an immoral, licentious woman, the golden girl of the age. Frigidity, it seemed, had entered her soul.

Miraculously, that young woman had suddenly awakened to her repressed natural desires. Hers was no furtive corner-and-whole liaison. The two friends visited people together, attended functions together, just wandered about together. They were happy to be seen together.

There was also a charming little detail about their friendship. The man was younger than Rukhmabai.

And he was no despicable fop and masher. He was aware that visiting France was, then in England, de rigueur to be a man, or woman, of culture. He certainly minded being taken for a 'black fellow', not even an Abyssinian prince. He was like any educated Indian of his day – the best of them – who claimed equality with their white rulers and, forgetting their own colour, denigrated Black Africans. Or like Lord Salisbury, the British prime minister, who derided Dadabhai Naoroji as a 'black man', unmindful that Naoroji was fairer than him.

Antoinette Burton speculates that the man was the 'Rajah of Kolapore'. No Rajah of Kolhapur would have condescended to enter the ICS. Tracing this friendship back to Bombay, Burton further speculates: 'Given that Nora Scott met both Rukhmabai and the Rajah in Bombay, it may well be that Rukhmabai knew him before she saw him in London.'[33] Nora's *Journal* mentions the Rajah only once to say: '... such a jovial, honest, friendly fellow. Mr Kemball brought him to me and introduced us. He knows him well, and likes him very much.'[34] Not even remotely does this relate to Rukhmabai.

The young man, whom Cornelia caricatured as Mutgatkar, was Govind Dinanath Madgavkar. Born in 1871, he graduated from the Elphinstone College, Bombay, before going to Balliol. A brilliant chess player who played on top board for Oxford in 1892, he was described by a contemporary authority on the game as having 'astonishing sight of the board, which enabled him to leave his own game and wander round, looking at others and passing acute comments on their prospects'. He did get into the ICS, rose to be a judge of the Bombay High Court, was knighted, and retired as a judge of the supreme court of Kolhapur.

Rukhmabai had no reason to be ashamed of her friend.

Govind left London in the middle of 1892 for his first posting in Burma. One can't be certain how much of the friendship survived London. But we do know that friendship with this adventurous, fun-loving, uncommonly talented youth brought into young Rukhmabai's sad life a joy and an abandon she would not know again. This gift, too, she owed to London. Were it not for the exhilarating freedom the city naturally provided, she could not have found that temporary release from her puritanic aversion to love and marriage.

What London made possible ended with London. Once back

home, she slipped into the life of loneliness to which law and custom had condemned her.

The pathos of this friendship is palpable. So is the animus against Rukhmabai that burst forth in Cornelia's vicious account of the friendship. That animus, moreover, points to a tragedy that afflicted Rukhmabai for no fault of hers and over which she had no control. Cornelia was one whom Rukhmabai had done her best to befriend. Encouraged by Elizabeth Manning, Rukhmabai had made an overture and written to Cornelia a letter of welcome even before she reached England on 19 September 1889. Wishing to bring the two gifted Indian girls together, Manning arranged for them to stay together in her house in the affluent neighbourhood of Maida Vale. The two girls even went about London and visited the stunning fifteenth-century Hampton Court Castle. Rukhmabai was utterly delighted; Cornelia 'was mad with despair and fatigue'. 'Rukhmabai,' she complained, 'is tired of nothing.'[35]

Rukhmabai had about her an aura that brought her immense admiration, sympathy and friendship. But, especially among the more ambitious and unconfident of her countrywomen, it also produced resentment, antipathy and rivalry. Rukhmabai never gave Cornelia Sorabji any offence. Yet, as noted by her nephew and biographer, Richard Sorabji, Cornelia viewed Rukhmabai as a rival and was 'uncharitably wary' towards her.[36] Antoinette Burton is more forthright. Describing Cornelia's 'cattiness' towards Rukhmabai, Burton writes: 'As time went on, Sorabji expressed more and more resentment toward Rukhmabai, quite possibly because Rukhmabai was pursuing the course of study [medicine] Sorabji herself desired.'[37]

The irrational hostility that seized Cornelia released its own force. There remained no objective limits to what she could imagine, believe and say about Rukhmabai. Cornelia could not stop at condemning what she saw as Rukhmabai's disgraceful behaviour in that one instance. She portrayed Rukhmabai as a woman of easy virtue and demeaned her crusade as a wilful woman's self-indulgence. Consumed by hostility, Cornelia also assailed Rukhmabai fatuously for 'wandering about most publicly alone' in the streets of London. She forgot that about the only time she had truly admired Rukhmabai was for travelling alone from London to Oxford to hear Lady Dufferin's lecture on medical aid for India, whereas Cornelia, as a student at Oxford's Somerville Hall, would not go unchaperoned even to her classes.

Rukhmabai did not let even the punishing pressure of medical studies wean her from public work on behalf of her British and Indian sisters. But after returning home she eschewed public activities and dedicated herself to service as a doctor. That decision was not unconnected with the realization that she was powerless to prevent the hostility she unwittingly aroused and the ensuant damage to the concerned cause. So complete was Rukhmabai's subsequent transformation that even Cornelia forgot her earlier disapprobation of Rukhmabai's involvement with the 'Women's Rights Women', and summed her up thus:

> An unusual and fine character and almost stolid ... Rukhmabai has returned as a doctor to India, and has served her country with ability and dignity ... Unemotional and untouched by the hysteria of politics or "Women's Rights".[38]

Another lasting friendship that Rukhmabai formed was with the women's rights activist and suffragist, Louisa Martindale, whom she met through Eva McLaren. They became close enough for Rukhmabai to spend some of her holidays at Louisa's home in Brighton. Louisa had two daughters, of whom the elder was named after the mother, Louisa, and the younger Hilda. They felt drawn to their mother's Indian friend and, to quote the elder one, admired her 'graceful figure in her brightly coloured sari, with charming manners and a keen sense of humour'. Louisa Jr became a doctor and rose to be an eminent surgeon. She, too, became friends with Rukhmabai. The Martindales, in turn, became Rukhmabai's guests in Surat.

Rukhmabai's swansong in the UK was an appeal for funds to promote Indian women's education. This was a cause she had espoused all through her six years' sojourn. As Hannah Whitall Smith put it: 'It is for this Rukhmabai is working.'[39] Whether it was a public meeting or an interview, she underscored the neglect of female education in British India. Towards the end of 1892, she – Bai Rukhmabai as she had begun to be addressed by the British press – even joined a high-powered deputation to present an influentially signed memorial to the Secretary of State for India, the Earl of Kimberley, and told him that only educated women could improve the condition of women in India.

Extensively broadcast by the British press, Rukhmabai's parting appeal said:

> From the depths of my own experience I would appeal to the English nation, who have already done so much for my country, to add to their other kindnesses this one that is so sorely needed by the women of India, who know not where else to turn for help. The education of Indian girls over ten years of age receives but little sympathy even from wealthy native gentlemen, and, of course, it is impossible to obtain money for such a purpose from the mass of the population. And the money with which I may be entrusted will be invested as a separate fund for aiding the English schools for native girls ... I therefore earnestly appeal to friends of the women of India to give their generous help, and so confer a great boon on Indian women.

The appeal was meant to raise money for the Students' Literary and Scientific Society of Bombay. Founded in 1848 by a group of brilliant young men, such as Naoroji Fardunji, Dadabhai Naoroji, Bhau Daji and S. S. Bengali, the Society was, at the time of Rukhmabai's appeal, headed by Justice M. G. Ranade and had among its members notables like Pherozeshah Mehta and Behramji Malabari. It possessed, Rukhmabai explained, the necessary organization but not the necessary funds. She would be happy with a subscription of 2,000 pounds sterling.

Besides aiding the education of her Indian sisters, Rukhmabai's appeal was also an expression of gratitude for the great support she had received during the difficult years of her trial. Malabari, Mehta and Ranade – all of them associated with the Students' Literary and Scientific Society of Bombay – had variously supported Rukhmabai during her trial. Her appeal was also an act of plain self-effacement, a trait that would define her entire life. Finally, the appeal was a reaffirmation of her faith in the British and their rule. That faith never deserted her.

8

Quiet Service

Rukhmabai returned to Bombay in January 1895. The very following month she was appointed House Surgeon at the Cama Hospital in place of Dr Freny Cama, who was proceeding on leave for a month. Just as that vacancy ended, Dr Sharp proceeded on privilege leave for six months and Cama was appointed locum for Dr Sharp. That got Rukhmabai an extension of six months. The seven months of the two successive leave vacancies finally ended in August.

But she was not one to remain jobless for long. Scarcity of Indian women doctors apart, she carried a surplus market value as an alumnus of the prestigious London School of Medicine for Women. She enjoyed, moreover, the backing of the most influential woman in the world of Indian medicine, Edith Pechey. If there was any uncertainty, it was about the kind of job the next one would be. Before the year was over, Rukhmabai found herself taking up residence in the bustling business city of Surat, just 175 miles from Bombay. She was appointed to head the upcoming Seth Morarbhai Vrijbhukhandas Hospital and Dispensary for Women and Children.

Professionally, she could not have asked for a better job. Seven months of a subordinate position in a large Bombay hospital had permitted her little scope for individual initiative. Holding independent charge of a hospital in a middle-sized, rich business city would give her the freedom to chart out her own path and put into practice the missionary spirit and philosophy of her alma mater, the London School of Medicine for Women. No less importantly, heading a new hospital would leave her untrammelled by the practices and conventions of any predecessors.

From a purely personal point of view also the Surat job was a great blessing. It enabled Rukhmabai to leave Bombay, and yet be within convenient distance from it. Bombay had, of course, accorded her a warm welcome on her return. But that had not ended the old hostility that her refusal to be a dutiful Hindu wife had brought upon her. There had even been attempts to excommunicate her for the sin of crossing the seas. However equanimous she might like to be, the persistence of the orthodox Hindu venom was a nuisance. Escaping the city brought her much psychological relief and peace of mind.

The foundation stone of the Surat hospital was laid on 5 November 1894 by the Governor of the Bombay Presidency, Lord Harris. This happened, coincidentally, barely two months before Rukhmabai's return from London, and the hospital started looking for its first doctor just when she was looking for a decent job. The coincidence was made possible by two larger developments away from Surat: the 'medical women for India' movement and the establishment of the Countess of Dufferin's Fund.

While women in Britain were not altogether averse to consulting male doctors, in cases involving the examination of their private parts, even they, with their inherited modesty and shyness, were loath to being seen by a male doctor. The situation in India was infinitely worse. Whatever the ailment, as Dr Hilda Lazarus observed, Indian women 'would suffer silently even to death rather than be examined by men'.[1] While this was generally true, male doctors were, in the event of serious ailments, occasionally called to treat women in families that could afford the expense. In such cases, however, the physician was not permitted a close, intimate examination. Other than *dais*, home remedies, prayers and supernatural practices, there was little to alleviate the misery of ailing women. To quote Hilda Lazarus again:

Even those who have come out of purdah or do not observe purdah, with their generations of inherited bashfulness, modesty and shyness, would still prefer hospitals staffed by women and attendance [sic] by women. It is not her false modesty, but her quiet, shy and bashful nature that sometimes makes it difficult for an Indian woman to relate her symptoms even to a female doctor. She generally pours out her tale of woe to her nearest woman relation or friend who is her spokeswoman. As long as this attitude of mind remains, and it is her privilege to choose her medical attendant, the need for women doctors in India will continue and not in the field of curative medicine alone, but in preventive medicine and in the uplift of humanity. The number of women's hospitals and women doctors are far too few to meet the growing demand for such.[2]

Women's suffering as a consequence of the neglect of their medical care – especially the egregious incidence of maternal and infant mortality – was hidden from no one. But, rather than be seen as preventable by human intervention, it was acquiesced in as 'the toll of Nature' and 'will of God'.

Christian missionaries were the first to intervene. Aiming to reach into the Indian zenana, they began in certain parts of India to employ female medical workers. However, most of those workers were barely trained to do medical work. Their incompetence apart, they were avoided also because of their connection with Christian missions and people's fear of proselytization.

Nevertheless, the situation was so dire that it also produced a nascent secular awareness of the need to provide women with physicians of their own sex. Soon a man of action with a burning sense of urgency appeared on the scene. This was a public-spirited American named George Kittredge (1833–1917). An entrepreneur making his money in Bombay, Kittredge was appalled that:

At this time there was no lady with a medical degree in the Bombay Presidency; in Bengal and the North-West there were one or two connected with the Missionary Societies. In Madras the same held true.[3]

In no time an influential group of the city's notable Indians came forward to help Kittredge. The most enthusiastic and resourceful of them was the eminent social reformer, Sorabjee Shapurjee Bengallee (1831–93). Coming together in 1882, Kittredge and Bengallee initiated what the *Times of India* aptly described as the medical women for India movement. Their first lasting achievement was to win for women the right of admission to medical colleges in India. They also inaugurated the Medical Women for India Fund of Bombay to raise money by public subscription. Within a mere four years they were ready with India's first hospital for women. This was the Cama Hospital, so named after Pestonji Hormusjee Cama, a Poona-based Parsi millionaire who, having promised a donation of one lakh rupees, ended up contributing a total of 1,64,300 rupees. Staffed and administered entirely by women, the Cama Hospital was independent of government interference and control. It was during its formative years headed by none other than Edith Pechey, whose importance in Rukhmabai's life we have already seen.

Within three years of the medical women for India movement's inauguration, the British Indian government, too, awoke to its responsibility. Their waking up was due to a combination of human and imperialist impulses. The human impulse related to the government's belated realization of its obligation to its suffering female subjects. The imperialist impulse was meant to mitigate the dangers of the gender war that had engulfed the medical 'fraternity' in Britain. W. W. Hunter candidly described it thus:

> As an outlet for qualified lady doctors, it suggests a solution of the problem as to how to freely throw open the British medical profession to the female sex, without unduly intensifying the hard struggle for life, which is already the lot of nine-tenths of the medical practitioners in this country [Britain].[4]

That led to the creation of the Countess of Dufferin's Fund in 1885. Raised with private donations, chiefly from the Indian princes, this was a quasi-official fund which possessed the prestige of connection with the government without being fully controlled by it. The Fund created a network of hospitals and dispensaries for women and children. But it did not treat female doctors as the equals of their male counterparts. Disregarding the Kittredge-Bengallee model, the Fund subordinated female doctors to male officials and paid them lower salaries.

The British Indian authorities recognized the importance of female doctors without being fair to them. Indifferent to their self-respect and material well-being, the authorities institutionalized the inferiority of female doctors to men. The slowly expanding community of female doctors would need decades to come together and wage a long struggle against gender discrimination.

The Countess of Dufferin Fund opened local branches all over the country. Its Surat branch, presided over *ex officio* by the District Collector, had Kalabhai Lallubhai as it first secretary. A lawyer by profession, Kalabhai was a progressive-minded public figure. As a student at Bombay's Elphinstone Institution, he had been taught by stalwarts like Dadabhai Naoroji and Principal Wordsworth. Promoting a variety of causes, he was particularly concerned about the neglect of women's health. Supported by his wife, Mahalakshmi,

Kalabhai took virtual charge of his city's branch of the Lady Dufferin Fund. Their good work was carried on by their son, Runjeetram Kalabhai, and daughter-in-law, Usha. The same age as Rukhmabai, Runjeetram and Usha became her friends and faithfully stood by her through the twenty-two years of her not-always-easy existence in Surat.

After over one lakh rupees had been locally raised, Mahalakshmi persuaded Lady Reay, wife of the governor of Bombay, to permit the Surat branch to utilize the money instead of sending it to the central fund. That done, Mahalakshmi and Kalabhai set about knocking at the city's many rich doors. They were enthused by the fact that, within just three years of Bombay's Cama Hospital, Gujarat, too, had got its first hospital for women and children. Called the Victoria Jubilee Hospital, it was built in Ahmedabad by Ranchhodlal Chhotalal, the father of the city's cotton textiles industry. Their knocking ended at the door of their city's best known philanthrope, Bai Dayakore.

Married as a twelve-year-old to Sheth Morarbhai Vrijbhukhandas, thirty-three years her senior, Dayakore was widowed in 1884 when she was thirty-eight. Though illiterate, she had so impressed the Sheth with her business acumen that he had willed his entire property to be managed by her. The philanthropic widow readily contributed ₹40,000 of her own and ₹36,000 from a legacy for charity that her late husband had bequeathed. She stepped in again a decade later to provide money for the hospital's expansion.

Thus came into being the hospital that brought Rukhmabai to Surat. Though it was opened to the public on 30 November 1896, Rukhmabai took charge a year earlier in October 1895. Edith Pechey, we may recall, had assumed charge of the Cama Hospital more than two years before it started functioning. The arrangement enabled Rukhmabai to fine-tune the building in keeping with the peculiar requirements of a hospital, and also furnish and equip it accordingly. She also chose the skeletal support staff of three with whom she, as the hospital's sole doctor, would serve the city's ailing women and children.

Rukhmabai, characteristically, did not wait for the hospital's completion to commence her medical work. Put up in a house belonging to the Kalabhais, she converted part of it into a makeshift dispensary and started treating patients.

The Morarbhai Vrijbhukhandas Hospital was a handsome two-storeyed stone structure in the busy city's noisy centre. The ground floor consisted of an outdoor dispensary, waiting room, consulting room, wards with accommodation for twenty indoor patients, and an office. On the first floor was the medical officer's modest apartment. In that apartment would be spent the rest of Rukhmabai's twenty-two years in Surat.

While coming to Surat, she was, naturally, apprehensive that the city's Hindus, remembering her as a disgrace to their society, might not take kindly to her. But the Surtis, true to their traditional liberal ethos, did not take long to accept her as a friend and benefactress. She – soon to become Bai to the locals – could not have asked for more.

Rukhmabai was already thirty. Having lived in two stepfamilies, an English home and a boarding house, she had not yet had a home of her own. Surat gave her that. She set it up with great love and care. It carried the same appearance of simplicity that marked her sartorial elegance. Further, it was unlike the typical Indian household where anyone claiming to be a relative or friend could descend and depart at will. Growing up in two stepfamilies had taught her what family life should not be. As against that, the memorable year at the McLarens and four years at the College Hall had given her certain clarity about how she would organize her family life. She would not accept unwanted guests.

There is a tantalizing cryptic description of Rukhmabai's home in Surat. This comes from Dr Margaret Ida Balfour. Visiting the city in her capacity as Secretary to the Dufferin Fund, she wrote that Rukhmabai 'lives over the hospital but quite in European style'. It is possible that Balfour's observation related to aspects of Rukhmabai's social life. It is also possible that Balfour saw something European in the setting up of the house, say, for dining, toilet and bathroom, etc. But in one respect, which Balfour could not have seen, her observation holds absolutely true. Rukhmabai made her home her castle.

She decided whom she would host inside the castle. Those she accepted were welcomed most warmly. She made them feel wanted and even organized entertainment for them. For example, when her old friend, women's rights activist and suffragist Louisa Martindale, and her two daughters were staying with Rukhmabai, she organized for them a mesmerizing performance by four jugglers. The jugglers brought with them snakes, including cobras and a mongoose. The many acts they performed included swallowing fire and the finale came by way of a fight between a cobra and the mongoose. Though this was part of the jugglers' normal repertoire, something abnormal happened that night, to the ladies' consternation. Carried away by the occasion and the lure of a fat *bakshish*, the jugglers let the fight continue until the mongoose had killed the cobra.

Hosting old friends like the Martindales made Rukhmabai supremely happy. However, they did not come frequently enough to mitigate the loneliness of her life. That was rather done by Rukhmabai's willingness to host some of her half-blood kin from her maternal grandfather and stepfather. The ones she particularly welcomed were the children of her siblings from her mother's marriage with Sakharam Arjun and the children of her mother's siblings from Harishchandra Yadavji's second marriage. Some of these kids came regularly and spent their vacations with Rukhmabai. She even took them to Dumas, a beach resort for rich Surtis at the mouth of the river Tapti, where she had rented a small house.

In 1897, within months of the hospital's formal opening, the plague epidemic broke out in Surat. Rukhmabai was given charge of the women patients at the Civil Hospital. As the pestilence raged on, she also had to undertake house-to-house visitation in the sprawling city to look for women and children affected by the disease. For nine gruelling months she knew no rest or respite. She was, during those trying days, sustained by the spirit of 'female professionalism' she had imbibed at the London School of Medicine for Women. What helped her professionally in coping with the pestilence was the knowledge she had acquired while doing that optional course on preventive medicine.

For her services during the plague, Rukhmabai was awarded the Kaisar-i-Hind Silver Medal by the British Indian government.

Only after the plague was over could Rukhmabai concentrate fully on her own hospital. Before turning to that, it will help to get an idea of the general atmosphere in which female doctors – particularly Indian female doctors – had to operate. The medical women for India movement, the Countess of Dufferin Fund and the founding in rapid succession of women's hospitals in Bombay, Ahmedabad and Surat manifested an awakening within both the Indian society and the colonial administration. These were welcome developments that gave a sense of self-worth to the intrepid female trespassers into the male bastion of medicine. But neither by the administration nor by society were those intrepid women treated with the dignity and respect they were entitled to.

Even as the government condemned them to institutionalized gender discrimination, the society behaved no better. Individuals apart, the society as a whole betrayed towards its pioneering medical women a blind, irrepressible hostility. Its hostility sprang from a deep-rooted conservatism that accepted as axiomatic the customary separation of the home and the outside, *ghare-baire* as Tagore memorably put it. The separation was believed to be essential to social order and morality. Over time an intricate web of mores, taboos and sanctions had evolved to keep that order and morality firmly in place. There obtained a collective mode of feeling and thinking that reacted with horror to any violation of that sacred separation. Built into that mode of feeling and thinking was an irrational – consequently the more uncontrollable – fear of women stepping out into the world outside. Such women, it was commonly feared, would wantonly throw open the floodgates of debauchery. That fear, in turn, aroused unrestrained anger against them.

This is reflected in the obscene slandering of India's first practising female doctor, Kadambini Ganguly (1861–1923). Reminiscent of the humiliating public portrayal of Rukhmabai as the golden girl of the age, Dr Ganguly was likened to a whore in *Bangabasi,* a leading periodical of Bengal. Not all the pioneering Indian women of medicine were so wildly vilified. But there was none who escaped public denunciation. Irrespective of its intensity in specific cases, at the heart of each denunciation lay the same complex of fear and anger.

Rukhmabai, too, had to bear her share of travails as a female doctor. But she was fortunate that what she had to endure was nothing in comparison to her coevals' ordeals. For one, she had already during her litigation suffered great ignominy and learnt to take it in her stride. More than that, she was lucky to have got a job in Surat. Going by Indian standards, Surat was an astonishingly permissive city, and its people were not so prone to visions of moral breakdown.

But that did not make the Surtis accepting of the outlandish phenomenon of women doctors. They, too, were disinclined to send their women to zenana hospitals. Rukhmabai had to work hard to make herself professionally accepted and trusted. She was lucky that just four months after her hospital started functioning, it was visited by the vicereine, Lady Elgin. The visit received prominent coverage in the press. Newspaper reports highlighted the fact that

Her Excellency, along with her party, which included Brigade-Surgeon Lt Col Franklin, was received and taken around the hospital 'by the Lady Physician, Miss Rukhmabai, M.D.'. There was in the reports special mention of the fact that the superintendence of Miss Rukhmabai had already within that short span turned the hospital 'into one of the most successful zenana charities in India'.

But, more than newspaper reports, it was word of mouth that filled the city with tales of how the 'England-returned' lady physician had by her exceptional dignity, grace and composure won over the vicereine and her party. There was a sudden upsurge in Rukhmabai's stock. She who could so parley with the Great Lady was not to be taken lightly or messed with.

The formidable impression thus created was deepened by the ease and naturalness with which Rukhmabai interacted with the white sahebs administering the district. While all Indians, not excluding the affluent local aristocracy, had their heads habitually bowed in deference to the sahebs, this Indian woman was a regular member of the sahebs' exclusive club and played tennis there with none other than the king of the district, the collector.

Rukhmabai, however, knew that the awe people felt for her would by itself do little to facilitate the work that had brought her to Surat. If anything, it could even stoke the irrational hostility they habitually felt towards an independent professional woman. She needed to reach out to people and inspire in them the trust that she was one of their own. That she had come to serve their women and children. She needed to induce people of all classes and communities to be easy and natural with her, like she was with the sahebs.

She directed all her qualities of head and heart to achieve this. She betrayed no superciliousness, impatience or exasperation on account of what her education and training made her view as people's ignorance and superstition. Rather, she applied all her powers of empathy to get under people's skin to try and understand their ways of thinking, feeling and behaving. Knowing that the surest way to people's hearts lies in their language, she learnt Gujarati quickly and soon was proficient in it.

As a female doctor in charge of a hospital for women and children, the maximum cases she had to treat related to gynaecology and obstetrics. To make the Western modes of pre-natal, natal and post-natal care acceptable, she had to neutralize the multiple quasi-religious customs and practices, with their attendant prescriptions and taboos, that different communities observed from the time of conception to birth and the days immediately thereafter. Some of those practices were patently unacceptable to the Western medical system.

To offer by way of illustration a practice that is still not extinct, a woman was believed to be in a state of impurity – *sutak* or *ashauch* – after giving birth to a child. She was put in isolation, usually in an unventilated dark room, for a prescribed period which could range to a maximum of forty-five days. This was a near-universal practice. Except among the poor labouring classes, which would not lose a new mother's wages for a day longer than was necessary. Rukhmabai often narrated the story of visiting a woman, whose child she had delivered the previous day. Wanting to see how that forceps case was progressing, she found the woman milking a cow. Though much less than the mother's unhygienic isolation during sutak, this, too, was a source of anxiety for Rukhmabai as a doctor.

There also were some other, less common and more peculiar, practices that she had to contend with. One such practice, which she narrated with great relish, related to a community in Saurashtra. The umbilical cord was not allowed to be cut in this community. The placenta was placed in an earthen pot and covered with ashes. The placenta had to be taken along whenever the baby was put to the breast.

So unpropitious, then, was the situation in Surat and even more so in Rajkot twenty-two years later, in which Rukhmabai had to earn respect and acceptance. She did that with great tact, patience and pragmatism. An obituary in the *World Medical Journal* summarized this aspect of her achievement. Saying that 'she was not impulsive but quietly observant', the obituary remarks that:

> instead of trying to bring about changes and thus antagonize the population, she worked tactfully and gradually spread the right ideas. Through her persistent efforts and energy, medical aid was carried to the remotest hut, where even forceps deliveries and other obstetric operations had to be performed on cowdung floors with only a flickering light burning; even water was difficult to obtain.[5]

Rukhmabai was equally patient and pragmatic in handling the traditional system of midwifery with its key actor, the hereditary *dai*. From the vantage point of Western medical care, the dai was seen as an unadulterated evil, and there was no end to the stories of their alleged criminal deeds. But Rukhmabai was balanced enough to realize the usefulness of dais. Even as she organized the training of female nurses along Western lines, she also arranged to familiarize the dais with the rudiments of Western midwifery.

She had learnt from having had to end her principled fight for women's rights with a compromise. Persuasion and accommodation, not confrontation, would be her way to serve the society.

There is a famous story that shows how innovative Rukhmabai was in her efforts to convince the sceptical Surtis that their women were safer with her than with their dais. Even after women started coming to her for consultation and treatment, there was great resistance to hospitalization for fear that evil spirits might possess them there. One day she spied a pregnant sheep that had strayed into the hospital and kept it back. The sheep delivered inside the hospital and people saw that, unharmed by any evil spirits, both the mother and the newborn were bouncing. Rukhmabai got the press to report the event and emphasize the safety of hospitalization.

By and by people began to shed their reservations and fear. The Parsis as a community did that fast. Converting the Hindus and the Muslims was a slower process and more difficult.

Rukhmabai knew that it was difficult to make an alien system of medicine acceptable to any community, especially to their women. She also knew that getting all the communities and classes together was, in her day, next to impossible. The easiest course in the circumstances would have been to try and woo some and, for the time being, not worry about the others. She, instead, adopted a two-pronged policy which soon earned her universal respect, acceptance and clientele. She employed her elite persona to make her place among the rich and the respectable. Once that happened, they began calling her home to treat and help their women deliver. At the same time, she visited the poor and the neglected in their remote huts and showed by example that she was there to serve them. That was enough for them to start going to her as outdoor patients and also for hospitalization.

Rukhmabai was soon Surat's best-loved and most respected person. To her alone were equally opened the city's bungalows and havelis and its humbler houses and huts.

It is easy to imagine the squalor in which Rukhmabai visited the city's poor and won them over. Not so the luxury of the city's rich. Dr Louisa Martindale offers us a peep into that luxury. While they were staying with Rukhmabai, she, her mother and sister were invited home by some of the city's notables including the begum of the Nawab of Surat. Louisa wrote:

The palace was huge, with a lake and fountain in the background. We were met at the foot of the steps by the Begum's son … He conducted us upstairs to the women's quarters … We were ushered into a huge room and the boy disappeared. The ceiling was low and covered with beautiful dark Moorish carving. The furniture was Moorish too, and there was a delightful large swing bed. There were twenty-eight windows along the front elevation and I don't know how many at the side … we were taken … into another large room at the back where the Begum and her daughter received us … She had a green gauze tinselled veil all over her head and body and four or five ear-rings in each ear.[6]

Rukhmabai was no doubt greatly helped by her endearing personal qualities in being accepted by all. But that acceptance would not have counted for much if she had failed to be seen as a great healer. Given her indifferent performance as a medical student, this was unlikely to happen. But Rukhmabai effected the unlikely, and people began to believe that she could perform miracles and bring the dying back to life. This is what the local correspondent of the *Times of India* reported:

In her hospital (it is usually known as Rukhmabai's Hospital) and wherever in the city women and children need her help and her skill, Rukhmabai is to be found relieving pain by her gentle touch, inspiring confidence by her quiet manner. Only last week a poor woman lay in her hospital at the point of death. Everybody thought she was dying; nobody ever expected her to recover. But Rukhmabai, though not herself hopeful, never relaxed her efforts. She ordered special serum from Bombay, she ceaselessly attended the case, and something like a miracle occurred. The apparently dying woman was slowly coaxed back to life and she is now out of danger and is speedily regaining strength. That is but one example of the good work Dr Rukhmabai is doing.[7]

People deified her.

But we are told nothing specific about Rukhmabai's medical skills. Fortunately an elaborate first-hand account of a daring operation performed by Rukhmabai, which had for more than a century lain buried in the pages of a scientific journal, came to my attention. This account shows that she was not only a fine physician but also a proficient surgeon. She was a complete doctor.

One day a weak and thin sixty-year-old Muslim woman was ushered into Rukhmabai's chamber in the Morarbhai Vrijbhukhandas Hospital. Though worn-out-looking, she was able to walk about by herself. Six months back she had begun having a slight pain in the left iliac region. Her abdomen had begun to increase and by the time she came for treatment it had grown to be thirty-six inches round the waist at the level umbilicus. She had no appetite and got two or three loose motions a day. Before the ailment set in, she was a well-built woman with perfect health. Married when quite young, she had mothered a total of nine children. She had her menopause when she was around forty-five.

Rukhmabai saw that the distention of the woman's abdomen was abnormal and it needed to be immediately operated upon. Also that this was a difficult surgery and it could throw up unanticipated complications. She thought it best to discuss the case with Major Bennett, the Civil Surgeon of Surat. Bennett approved of her line of action and even agreed to assist Rukhmabai. The operation, however, was performed by Rukhmabai with Bennett by her side to aid her. Subsequently, when they felt that the case deserved to be brought to the notice of the medical community at large, Rukhmabai's name, following standard protocol, appeared as the senior author of their joint research paper.

The patient, having expressed her willingness to be operated upon, was hospitalized on 5 July 1907. The technical intricacies of the operation may be difficult for lay readers to follow. But it is best to record them so as to convey a sense of Rukhmabai's skill as a surgeon.

The woman's abdomen was distended vertically from ensiform cartilage to pubes, and laterally from flank to flank. There was no variation of note from change of position. It was dull all over, though thrill was elicited on tapping the abdomen simulating fluid. No hard masses could be felt. The skin was tense and shining over the abdomen.

The operation was performed on 12 July. The patient was anaesthetized and a three-inch-long vertical incision was made in the middle line between the umbilicus and pubes. After the peritoneum was cut through, a bluish-black-looking mass protruded out of the wound, which was taken for the sac of the cyst; no fluid came out as expected. But when it was removed, thick jelly-like stuff welled up.

Later, during the operation, the incision was enlarged and the sides of the abdomen were pressed together and the jelly-like stuff was scooped out by the hand. Each handful brought out a thick calf's-foot-jelly-like substance. The substance sometimes looked bluish-white and opaque, and sometimes of watercolour transparency. In parts its contents were as thick and inelastic as kneaded dough.

The substance was such that it could not be removed entirely. It was filling every nook and corner of the abdominal cavity up to the diaphragm and down to the pelvic fossae. In parts it seemed to grow from the inner surface of the parietal peritoneum, and from there it extended in stalactite formation to the cyst wall and to the intestine coils. The cyst was very thin and adherent to the peritoneum in front. Both had blended together and were so easily lacerated that separation from one another was impossible and portions of the sac had to be left behind.

When the abdominal cavity was emptied of its jelly-like contents, it was found that the cyst had originally started from the right ovary, and as it went on increasing in size, the cyst got adherent to the peritoneum. However, the pedicle in the right broad ligament was carefully tied and a sac weighing over two pounds was removed. This part of the cyst was full of a number of small and pendicular cysts containing the same substance.

The whole quantity of the semi-fluid substance removed filled a pail of three and a half gallons.

The abdominal cavity was washed out with pints of warm distilled water to float up the jelly and facilitate its removal. A glass drainage tube was put in at the lower end of the incision and the wound closed with interrupted sutures.

The patient collapsed at this stage and seemed on the point of going off, but rallied in a short time.

The following three days she was in a rather low condition. Her temperature varied between 100 and 102, and the pulse was low between 90 and 100. There was also retention of urine. On the fourth day the tube was removed and a couple of sutures were put in to close the opening.

The woman was kept on slop diet for a week, then on light solid food. There was no fever or any other complaint after the fourth day. The stitches were removed on the tenth day. The wound had healed by first intention. The patient's recovery was uninterrupted. She was discharged from the hospital, feeling quite well, on 12 August, exactly a month after the operation.

The story does not end with the operation. Post-surgery, Rukhmabai did not go about celebrating her success. Sensing that a new discovery was in the offing, she continued her consultations with Dr Bennett and studied the processes underlying the ever-growing tumour. A specimen of the jelly-like stuff from the operated patient's abdomen was sent to the Parel Laboratory, Bombay, and the tumour was found to be a myxoma. After considerable reflection, Rukhmabai, aided by Bennett, did come up with a new discovery. Following Herman's standard *Diseases of Women*, there obtained at that time two theories about the origin of such a growth. One, that it sprang from an original tumour, either from a bit left behind after the tumour had been operated upon, or from some of its tissues that had got into the peritoneum owing to tapping or rupture. The other, that it was a growth of the peritoneum.

But here was a growth that neither of the prevailing theories could explain. It was not a bit of an original tumour that had been left behind by an operation or pushed into the peritoneum as a result of tapping or rupture. None of those procedures had taken place in this case. Nor was this a growth of the peritoneum – for there was a distinct pedicle and sac originating from the broad ligament. Instead, Rukhmabai and Bennett suggested that:

> the ovarian growth was myxomatous from the beginning, that the cyst wall being adherent to the general peritoneum, the latter became secondarily involved by the myxomatous tissues which grew along it and between the coils of the intestines.

Finally, cautious as any sensible researcher ought to be, Rukhmabai and Bennett avoided making any unwarranted claims, and concluded:

> The period since the operation has been too short to pronounce an opinion as to the probability of recurrence. The woman is at present in good health and able to perform satisfactorily all her household duties.[8]

The operation, seen in the context of the state of medical advance at the time, bears eloquent testimony to Rukhmabai's qualities and skills as a surgeon. She evidently possessed an uncanny diagnostic ability to read the symptoms and history of a case. She could discern the subtlest of signs and see what lesser doctors would most likely miss. This enabled her to anticipate what she would encounter inside her sixty-year-old patient's distended abdomen. The same ability also helped her anticipate – and be ready for – the difficult surprises that could crop up once the Pandora's box was opened. This is exemplified in the way she read the related symptoms of 'shifting dullness' and 'thrill' to anticipate what awaited her inside the distended abdomen. She could not be certain, she sensed, whether ascites – fluid – or a growth would confront her there. She was ready for both.

Further, Rukhmabai's determination to perform the difficult operation showed that she also possessed such other essential attributes of a good surgeon as self-confidence, courage and readiness to take risks. Above all, inside the operation theatre she showed with the scalpel the same suppleness of wrists which she had shown on the tennis court in London. She retained her cool when the patient collapsed and all seemed over. To cap all these qualities, she had the sense and the humility to seek consultation and assistance from the one doctor in the city whom she considered worth consulting.

That was no mean achievement. As a rule, female doctors with their supposed feeble wrists were in those days not expected to excel as surgeons. They were considered excellent if, apart from their routine duties as obstetricians, they could undertake minor operations. Even at a premier institution like the London School of Medicine for Women, we have seen, female students' training in surgery was not designed to equip them for much more.

The famous but indifferent student of the London School of Medicine for Women had made incredible strides within a mere ten years of being on her own as a doctor. She had blossomed into a fine physician, skilled surgeon and inquisitive researcher. And she always remained what she instinctively was: an ever-caring human being.

Evidence of this can be found in an anecdote that Louisa Martindale deemed worth recording for posterity. Rukhmabai, it so happened, received her first fee for an operation when the Martindales were staying with her. The fee, Louisa noted with an exclamation mark, was '4 annas!'

That royal fee, it appears from Louisa's narration, was announced by Rukhmabai to her British guests with much self-mocking fanfare, causing the four ladies to have a good laugh. Actually there was more to the fee than mirth and banter. Related to it was the sensitive issue of the dignity and status of female doctors. The issue is best understood by focusing on a controversy that was sparked off by Rukhmabai's friend and model, Edith Pechey. Gladly treating the patients gratis at the hospital, Pechey insisted on charging the same fee for a home visit as was paid to the city's best male doctors. That was ten rupees, forty times Rukhmabai's first fee for an operation. Insistence on getting ten rupees was for Pechey a matter of principle, not money. Accepting less, she said, would be tantamount to accepting the inferiority of female to male doctors. Her demand was seen as a betrayal of the ideal of service that she, as a doctor, was supposed to uphold. S. S. Bengallee, the great promoter of medical care for women, felt betrayed and severed all connection with the Cama Hospital. But Pechey was unmoved. She would readily, she said, visit a needy patient who could not afford the high fee and not charge a pie. But she would not accept less.

Rukhmabai admired Pechey and understood her mentor's refusal to budge on the question of female doctors' parity with their male counterparts. Rukhmabai herself was no less zealous about safeguarding the dignity of female doctors. In this regard, in fact, she had to wage a struggle that was even more difficult than Pechey's. As a woman belonging to the ruling race, Pechey had to struggle for parity only with male doctors. For Rukhmabai, an Indian woman who had dared to become a doctor, the struggle was not only vis-à-vis male doctors but also vis-à-vis European doctors who believed themselves to be superior to their Indian counterparts.

But she also knew that linking her dignity as a female doctor to the fee she charged would hurt the very women she had come out to serve. For, let alone the poor, even well-off Indians were loath – except perhaps in an emergency – to spend on calling a doctor for their ailing women. Rukhmabai, perforce, had to think of other ways to safeguard her position and dignity as a woman doctor. Like she did at the time of the difficult myxoma operation. Rather than play the second fiddle to the white civil surgeon – which is what colonized Indians routinely did in the presence of their alien masters – she led the operation and, following it, also the research that led to their joint paper.

While appointing Rukhmabai, the management of the Morarbhai Vrijbhukhandas Hospital could not have realized that they were making a dream appointment. They realized the difficulties of the charge they were entrusting the young woman with, and did not, realistically, expect her to overcome those challenges so quickly and with such consummate skill.

Except for the difficulty of financial constraints, which harassed Rukhmabai all along. It was clear from the outset that the hospital would need subscriptions to keep it going. What was not clear, not to Rukhmabai at any rate, was that subscriptions would be frustratingly elusive. On the contrary, the scenario looked most propitious in the beginning. The boss of the district, the collector and chairman of the committee that administered the hospital, constantly appealed to the Surtis for donations. He impressed upon them the importance of the hospital, their good luck in having got a doctor with the qualifications and energy of Rukhmabai, and their tradition of public charity. Visiting official dignitaries, too, would remind the locals of their obligation to the hospital. The press kept issuing its own intermittent exhortations.

Surat's reputation for charity was not misplaced. Affluent Surtis, indeed, gave freely. They gave to ensure a happy hereafter and also for gains here and now. They, besides, adored the lady doctor and were prolific in their admiration, encouragement and assurances. Young Rukhmabai was convinced that she had ended up in the right city.

Disillusionment awaited her. It set in when the hospital's need for fresh funds acquired urgency. The hospital, we may recall, had begun with a ward providing for a maximum of twenty indoor patients. That provision had then appeared prodigal. Even the poor, with their innate antipathy to Western medicine and fear of ghosts, would not hospitalize their women. But so remarkable was the turnaround effected by Rukhmabai that in less than ten years it became necessary to plan for a separate twenty-bed obstetric ward. The increased demand was primarily caused by pregnant women preferring to deliver in the hospital and not, as was customary, at home. The hold of the traditional dais was weakening.

A separate obstetric ward was indispensable. But that required money, and none was forthcoming. The same shetyas who had been so prolific with words would give nothing. They would give nothing for pure altruism, and never if their charity benefited an institution that commemorated another family. Their determined parsimoniousness comes through in the following report: 'Whilst Government, the Municipality, and the Local Board give fairly generous support to her [Rukhmabai's] hospital, only Rs 400 was received last year as "donations" and the whole of that sum came from the patients themselves.' The hospital, the report continued, practised 'every possible economy', and yet could not cover a deficit of Rs 350.[9] Furthermore, the boss of the district would not go beyond routine appeals and nudge a reluctant rich man to give.

In the midst of all the city's riches, Rukhmabai had none but the original donor to turn to. But even with Dayakore, Rukhmabai was not ready to take any chances. Unsure if she alone could pull it off with the old dowager, she sought help from her old friends Runjeetram and Ushaben. Through their good offices she persuaded Dayakore, who was then in Bombay, to salvage yet again the hospital named after her late husband. Dayakore, in a last act of munificence, promised a sum of 50,000 rupees. The money, she assured, would be released after she returned to Surat. But before she could return, Dayakore died in Bombay on 20 July 1904.

Childless Dayakore had in her will named as her successors Tribhovandas Narottamdas Malvi, Manubhai Rangildas Malvi and Natvarlal Maganlal Malvi. It was now up to these new masters of the Malvi fortunes whether to believe that their deceased aunt had, indeed, promised the donation, and to release the money promptly to expedite the construction of the ward. They believed, but dilly-dallied. They had their own priorities, politics and calculations. There was little for them, individually or collectively, to gain from releasing the money.

Reflecting their callousness – and the scale of Rukhmabai's difficulties – the three men procrastinated for eight and a half years. Meanwhile, in a subtle move to shift attention from Dayakore and Morarbhai Vrijbhukhandas, they got the family name 'Malvi' informally added to the hospital which hitherto had been known plainly as Morarbhai Vrijbhukhandas Hospital. Hoping thereby to acquire wider currency for the expanded name, they used their influence to get the press to describe the hospital as Morarbhai Vrijbhukhandas Malvi Hospital. Instead, people started calling it Rukhmabai's hospital. They still do.

Finally, on 21 January 1913, the foundation stone of the long-deferred new obstetric ward was laid by Sir Richard Lamb, Vice President of the Council of the Governor of Bombay. The ceremony was organized with great fanfare by Dayakore's successors who used it to claim credit for the Malavi family and for themselves. Speaking on the occasion, Tribhovandas Narottamdas Malvi, a flourishing solicitor, speculator and public figure, detailed the family's role in setting up the hospital, and told the assemblage how he and the other two successors of Dayakore had 'cheerfully agreed' to carry out her 'unwritten wishes'. He had little to say about Rukhmabai. That, significantly enough, was done by the Collector of Surat, Anderson, who spoke glowingly of her contribution to the hospital.

She was, indeed, the one who had brought the hospital to a point where, from struggling to attract patients, it was in need of expansion. It was also she who had been a mute witness to the systematic neglect of that need.

The foundation-laying ceremony ended Rukhmabai's growing frustration over the new ward's non-construction. However, the cheer that came with the ceremony proved false. The entire Morarbhai Vrijbhukhandas Hospital was built in under two years. The only sign of the new ward after two years was its foundation stone. Rukhmabai's frustration was back. So was her realization of being trapped in a situation she could do nothing to mend.

She escaped the trap on 1 October 1917. She was succeeded at the Morarbhai Vrijbhukhandas Hospital by Dr MRD Naoroji, another Edinburgh licentiate and a granddaughter of Dadabhai Naoroji.

Received accounts of Rukhmabai's Surat sojourn notice nothing odd here. The inordinate delay in the construction of the obstetric ward, which commenced with Dayakore's dying donation in 1904, is attributed to the World War of 1914–18. The strange disregard for chronology apart, it is not as if all construction activity had ceased during the war years. In any case, this construction was related to public health, which was a top priority even during the war. The hospital itself, in its appeal for funds during those years, was announcing that 'an obstetric ward with 20 beds is about to be added to the hospital'.

To miss the oddity of Rukhmabai's departure from Surat is to miss the underlying sadness of her life. Taking 1865 as the year of her birth, she was only fifty-two at the time of leaving the hospital which, as its first superintendent, she had single-handedly nurtured and developed. Fifty-two was well before the usual retirement age, and she had by then served the hospital for only twenty-two years. As against that, Motibai Kapadia, the first superintendent of the Victoria Jubilee Hospital in Ahmedabad, remained at the helm for the hospital's first forty years.

Rukhmabai's premature departure is telling. We must pause and listen to what it tells. So far we have not. We have either not noticed the oddity of the departure or seen it as a normal occurrence. Varde, for example, would have us believe: 'As per rules, she had to retire from the Surat hospital.' Reporting that all was well, Varde adds: 'Before retiring she drew up plans for enhancing the efficiency of the hospital and started a drive to collect funds for the same.'[10]

We can see that Rukhmabai's days at the Morarbhai Vrijbhukhandas Hospital, like her days at Sakharam's, have been memorialized as happy and harmonic. The reality of the days at Sakharam's, we have seen, was different. So was the reality of her two decades with the Surat hospital. The first of those decades was, in many ways, satisfying. That was when, overcoming difficult odds, she made herself and her hospital acceptable. In that acceptance lay her most significant achievement. She brought about, across the board, a new awareness about women within the family and about the family's obligation to them, particularly in the matter of their physical well-being. The more that awareness spread, the larger became people's acceptance of Rukhmabai and her hospital; so large as to necessitate the hospital's expansion.

Then things began to change, impressing upon her the futility of staying on. That happened by way of undercurrents of which the Surtis at large had no inkling. Only two years before she quit the Morarbhai Vrijbhukhandas Hospital, the local correspondent of the *Times of India* gushed:

'Rukhmabai!' Who does not know Rukhmabai? For the past 20 years she has been a familiar figure in the ancient city of Surat. There are, no doubt, other Rukhmabais – many of them – in the city, but there is only one Rukhmabai. Everybody knows who Rukhmabai is. She is one of the present possessions that we are proud of, that we glory in. We feel that if she should ever by any chance be removed from our midst the city would not and could not be the same without her and that a great gap – a gap that would be well-nigh impossible to fill – would be left. Rukhmabai is a doctor – a lady doctor – and she is every inch a lady and an out-and-out gentlewoman.[11]

This story carries no apparent hint that the city's beloved doctor might depart soon, much sooner than her scheduled retirement. It can be, though, read in two ways. One, considering newspersons' nose for, especially unsavoury, behind-the-scene goings-on and their papers' appetite for such stories, it is plausible that the situation was tolerable till at least the end of 1915; that a breakdown occurred during the intervening two years. The story also warrants a diametrically opposite reading. It may as well have come from a knowing correspondent who was anxious to pre-empt the dreaded eventuality by broadcasting the lady doctor's indispensability to the city.

Irrespective of what lay behind the *Times of India* story, it is evident that Rukhmabai was forced out of the hospital to which she had given her all.

She left Surat to take charge of the Rasukhanji Zenana Hospital in the claustrophobic wilderness of princely Kathiawad. A self-respecting and dignified woman, she had imbibed the Western ethos during her years in Bombay and the UK. She could have been under no illusion that the petty tyrants ruling over the myriad Kathiawadi states and their ranis would ever deign to have with her anything remotely resembling the easy, non-obsequious relations she had with the British Indian rulers and their wives.

Legend has it that the Maharani of Palitana talked Rukhmabai into leaving Surat. The Maharani, it is said, assured Rukhmabai that the Palitana palace would be like home to her and she would also have her tennis there. The legend strains our credulity. Rukhmabai would be based a whole hundred miles away from Palitana, in Rajkot where the Rasulkhanji Hospital was. Moreover, Palitana was but one among the 200-odd princely states in Kathiawad, and she would need to answer calls from all of them. Her only protection would come from the fact that the hospital she was going to head was founded and administered by the British Indian authorities. But that would not protect her from the whims and hubris of the rajas and ranis of the states she would of necessity visit.

Rukhmabai deserved better than the ignominy of being forced out of the hospital and the city she had made her own and devotedly served. Adversities going as far back in her life as she could remember, she had taught herself to remain unvexed by them. But this one hurt profoundly. Leaving Surat was a cruel severance.

Rukhmabai had not only set up home in Surat. She had made the city her own. Apart from providing medical care to the city's women and children, she had made herself available to those who needed guidance in domestic and social matters. She had taken under her wings many of the city's young widows. One such widow was Shivagauri, the younger sister of the famous chemist and entrepreneur, T. K. Gajjar. Encouraged and guided by Rukhmabai, Shivagauri acquired sufficient self-confidence to start a home for widows – 'Vidhavashram' – in collaboration with another young widow, Bajigauri. Also, realizing that the little children of her poor indoor patients were left unattended, she started in the hospital premises an afternoon school for those children, and even taught there.

Rukhmabai had also started a lecture scheme for the women of Surat. This involved raising funds for the purpose and getting in touch with prospective speakers. In 1907, when the annual session of the Indian National Congress was held in Surat, she associated herself with the all-India women's conference, which was organized as a fringe activity of the Congress. It is noteworthy that she did this in spite of her avoidance of large public activities in general and of politics in particular. She did so primarily because the women's conference was presided over by Ramabai Ranade, whom Rukhmabai had admired for long and we have met in chapter one.

Just three or four years separating them, both Ramabai Ranade and Rukhmabai were exceptional women. It gave them great joy to be together and talk about things that mattered to both of them. But they were also appalled by the depths to which nationalist politics descended with a shoe being hurled at an opponent at the Surat Congress.

It was from Surat that, in 1908, Rukhmabai had got a chance to visit Europe. We have, as for so much about her life, no details of the Europe visit. Except for one sad fact. She had planned to cross the English Channel and spend some time in dear England and look up old friends. The one she was most looking forward to meeting was Edith Pechey. But, unfortunately, Pechey died on 14 April 1908. We have this from Rukhmabai:

> From her deathbed she wrote, on my recent arrival in Europe, begging me to land at Folkestone and visit her, and it will be an everlasting grief to me that she was gone, alas! before I reached England.

Leaving Surat, it bears reiteration, was a cruel severance.

Whatever her hurt and disappointment – maybe to get over that – Rukhmabai buried herself in work immediately upon reaching Rajkot. She took charge of the Rasulkhanji Hospital – also known as the Zenana Hospital – in the first week of October. In the first week of December, which was a mere two months later, she launched a three-year course of training in nursing and midwifery. That was meant to address the 'long-felt want of trained nurses and midwives in Rajkot and elsewhere in serious obstetric cases'. Soon her hospital was sending out eight to ten trained nurses every year.

Even as Rukhmabai was beginning to settle in her new job there occurred a weird repetition of history. Like the outbreak of the plague in Surat within months of the opening of the Morarbhai Vrijbhukhandas Hospital, Kathiawad was overrun by the influenza epidemic soon after Rukhmabai took charge in Rajkot. She was, as a result, saddled with the additional work of looking after segregation camps and hospitals in and around Rajkot. Recognizing her services during the epidemic, the government added a bar to her Kaisar-i-Hind medal.

Once normalcy was restored, Rukhmabai returned to the old pattern of her professional life. This, in effect, meant that along with performing her job as the head of the Zenana Hospital, she also busied herself with other useful schemes. She had grown up in a culture which had its generationally transmitted home remedies for everyday ailments, and people's dependence on professional doctors was minimal. That cultural experience was differently reinforced by what she learnt of the underlying philosophy of preventive medicine at the London School of Medicine for Women. She knew that the medical profession might never achieve its supreme ideal – making its own existence unnecessary – that Dr Helen Webb had talked about in her inaugural lecture at the School. But its practitioners could at least work towards maximizing the profession's redundancy. It was this urge to make people medically self-reliant that led Rukhmabai to popularise 'First Aid'. She delivered, along with one Captain Masurekar, a series of lectures at Rajkot's Male and Female Training Colleges to bring home the importance of 'First Aid'. Also, she associated herself with the newly established Red Cross in Kathiawad.

Besides undertaking ancillary medical activities, Rukhmabai also kept up her efforts to improve the condition of adversely circumstanced women, such as widows and victims of domestic abuse. These for her were no two discrete activities. For example, the nursing course she started immediately upon joining the Rasulkhanji Hospital was primarily meant to address the shortage of trained nurses. But she encouraged women in distress to join the course, disabused the trainees of received notions of women's inferiority, and inspired them to aspire to a life of freedom, self-reliance and dignity.

Rukhmabai had long back given up on large organized movements and directed her social service efforts to her immediate surroundings. In grateful remembrance of what women like Edith Pechey and Eva McLaren had so selflessly done for her, she did her best to help the deserving. Her method was to organize localized schemes that would bring together small groups, watch them closely and take the promising ones under her wings.

We have, courtesy Mohini Varde, information about two women – Bapuba and Vidyalakshmi – whom Rukhmabai spotted early and guided all along. Bapuba was a young widow who did the nursing course, joined the Rasulkhanji Hospital, and so excelled in her job as to start assisting Rukhmabai in conducting operations. Bapuba was so kind-hearted that she began looking after an 'illegitimate' girl who was born in the hospital and abandoned by her mother. Rukhmabai fully supported Bapuba's action, participated in raising the girl and arranged her marriage to a solicitor from a respectable family.

Vidyalakshmi was a young woman who had fled domestic violence and returned to her natal home where her self-respect would not let her stay indefinitely. She sought Rukhmabai's guidance. That led to Vidyalakshmi qualifying as a nurse and being appointed to the Rasulkhanji Hospital, where she became a key assistant of Rukhmabai in running not only the hospital but also the Red Cross and the 'First Aid' programme.

Bapuba and Vidyalakshmi, for their part, did their best to assist Rukhmabai. They sensed that running the hospital and attending to outstation calls was taking a heavy toll on her. They took it upon themselves to keep the hospital functioning while Rukhmabai was away on call.

Yet, there were limits to what Rukhmabai's dedication, combined with the dedication of her select staff, could do. In Rajkot, too, like in Surat, chronic shortage of funds frustrated her plans and efforts. Here, too, she was reduced to sending out appeals for funds that elicited little response. Mirroring the Surat shetyas' refusal to give for a hospital that commemorated another shetya and his family, Kathiawad's egomaniacal princes would not aid a hospital that perpetuated the philanthropy of Rasulkhanji, the Nawab of Junagadh.

Actually the situation in Rajkot was way more daunting. The area of her operation in Kathiawad was much larger. She was often required to be away from Rajkot on calls from Kathiawad's myriad states, and travelling within the vast region was difficult. That made the discharge of her duties physically draining. It also adversely affected the hospital's functioning, especially so far as the in-patients and emergency cases were concerned.

The only solution was to appoint a lady doctor to assist Rukhmabai. But – further evidencing that Rukhmabai had left Surat under duress – it was hard to attract female doctors to Kathiawad, and harder to retain them. For example, for three years in a row – 1926–28 – the Rasulkhanji Hospital advertised for the post of an Assistant Lady Doctor. The salary offered was a decent 150 rupees per month plus free quarters. For the first two years, either no suitable candidate was found or the appointee left soon. It meant that for two years in a row Rukhmabai had to make do without an assistant.

According to Mohini Varde, a total of five assistant lady doctors came to the Rasulkhanji Hospital during the thirteen years that Rukhmabai was there, and none of them stayed long. The descriptions we have of the five doctors further point to the difficulty of attracting good doctors to Rajkot; they also show how fortunate Rajkot and Kathiawad were in getting Rukhmabai. One of them was a Parsi convert to Christianity who, unmindful of the spectacle she made of herself, would go to the hospital riding a horse, with her dog in tow. She also played the truant and went out to see friends during hospital hours. Openly insubordinate, she even tried to prevail upon the British agent in Rajkot to dismiss Rukhmabai. He, instead, sent her packing.

Another, who came from the Andaman Islands, was described by Rukhmabai thus:

> Oh! My God! She was quite mad. She felt that whoever was looking at her was spitting at her. She felt that all her enemies had come chasing her from the Andamans and were now spitting at her. She even used to kick servants in the hospital. Naturally, I could not ask her to distribute medicines. We had to remove her after six months.

Of the third, Rukhmabai said:

> After nearly two years, we got a doctor from the Agra Medical College. Most of her time was spent in changing her saris, which was three to four times in a day. On Sundays, she wore saris with gold and silver border linings. She seemed more concerned about her appearance than about examining her patients. Once she committed an unpardonable mistake while mixing medicines for a patient, which resulted in exactly the opposite of the desired result. Thankfully, she herself resigned after a month, saying that life in Rajkot was very boring.

The fourth – a lady doctor working in a ladies' hospital! – left in disgust because she felt uncomfortable examining women's private parts. The last one, a rich local Parsi woman, was an inveterate investor who would not assist even in minor surgeries.[12]

Thus, no matter whether she had doctors to assist her or not, all through her stay in Kathiawad, Rukhmabai had to cope virtually single-handedly with the growing medley of in-patients, out-patients and outstation patients. Add to this physical toll her dreary social life in Rajkot, and we realize how cruel the severance from Surat was. The rich of Surat had, no doubt, kept their purses closed to her hospital; but they had opened their hearts and homes to her. In sharp contrast – barring some like Palitana – the petty autocrats of Kathiawad and their women would not deign to meet Rukhmabai the way she wished to be met, as an equal. Neither Rukhmabai's professional dedication nor the magnetism of her personality could break through their hauteur. Even the most famous of them all, one best exposed to the West, the cricketer-prince K. S. Ranjitsinhji, was no different. She could not demand that she be treated as an equal. But she could maintain a dignified distance. Which is what she did. It rankled.

Rukhmabai's isolation in Rajkot was further aggravated by her realization that the British serving there – predominantly army officers with their impregnable hauteur – were markedly different from those she had known in Bombay, Surat and, of course, back in the UK. She preferred to do without the pleasant social life – including her evening tennis – she had enjoyed in Surat through her association with the city's European gymkhana, politely declining the good offices of the few European officials who wanted to get her access to their exclusive club.

As for the city's notable Indians, Rukhmabai found only a few worth interacting with. One such was Sitaram Narayan Pandit. The same age as Rukhmabai, this man of refined taste and culture was an eminent lawyer who had studied law in England. He lived like a European in a sprawling double-storied bungalow with many stables. He employed a European governess for his daughters and sent his son, Ranjit, to be educated and qualify for the bar in England. But what most endeared Sitaram to Rukhmabai was his avid interest in tennis. He had three tennis courts in his bungalow! Foregoing access to Rajkot's European gymkhana was not quite the deprivation it would have been without Sitaram and his tennis courts.

Rajkot could never be home to Rukhmabai. Years in that unwelcoming city and region inured her to a diminished social existence. This stark difference, sadly, has remained unnoticed. Offering, typically, an undifferentiated account of her career as a doctor, the otherwise informed obituary in the *World Medical Journal* wrote:

> Dr. Rukhmabai worked in these district towns at a time when work by medical women was poorly appreciated and single-handed work by medical women far from safe for their person. But Dr. Rukhmabai evinced such courage and integrity in her work that ere long members of every community respected her and sought her advice and guidance even in domestic matters and family difficulties. Her popularity was immense both at Surat and at Rajkot.

The praise for Rukhmabai is not misplaced. The equation of Surat and Rajkot clearly is. Marked since birth for a life of void and sadness, the only time she felt full, free and happy was in the UK. Returning home, life was as before during the year in Bombay. Then, luckily, Surat brought her some semblance of respite. Rajkot failed to provide even that. If anything, the city aggravated her innate existential indifference. She, it seems, decided to give in once and for all. A gift she made in 1926 would suggest that. Coming after she had been a decade in Rajkot and four years before her retirement, the gift suggests that she had started preparing for a quiet, isolated existence. In the January of 1926 were opened the King Edward Memorial Hospital and the Seth Gordhandas Sundardas Medical College in Bombay. Rukhmabai donated all her sixty bound volumes of the *British Medical Journal* to the new College.

On the face of it, this may seem a normal happening. Rukhmabai had been in harness for thirty-odd years and would continue for another four years. Nevertheless, she needn't have retired when she did. She was around sixty-five at the time, and in good health. Even if it were to treat people gratis, she could have easily set up her own clinic and continued to work for some more years. Instead, she chose *vanaprastha*. Even though she settled in Bombay, she moved into the house she had built for herself. There she had the freedom to keep her kin as far or near as she pleased.

For the twenty-five years that she lived after retirement – momentous years in the life of her country – she kept herself scrupulously sequestered from happenings around her. There was something irrevocable about her decision to turn her back on public life and refrain from any potentially fractious organized activity. She even let alone the issue of male superiority in her profession. Thus, she kept out of the Association of Medical Women in India which was formed in January 1907 to promote female doctors' interests. The Association was formed in Bombay at a meeting held at the Cama Hospital, and Rukhmabai could easily have come down from Surat. Her priorities were very different.

But she happily joined the Bombay branch of the Association of British University Women in India. We know that she travelled to Bombay to attend the eighth annual dinner of the Association on 5 March 1923 at the elite Willingdon Sports Club. Twenty of the Association's forty-nine registered members, representing seven British universities, were present. The proceedings began with a toast to the King-Emperor, which was proposed by the Association's president, Mrs Sowerby, followed by the health of the guest, Lady Tata, being proposed by Mrs Hingeley. The dinner ended with a vote of thanks to the hostess, Mrs G. B. Thomas, which was proposed by Rukhmabai. Though we have information only about the dinner of 1923, it is likely that she had joined the Association from its inception and participated in its activities regularly. She cherished her British academic connection. That was reason enough for her to neither flaunt it nor seek any advantage from it.

9

Widow's Garb

ONE DAY A TELEGRAM REACHED Rukhmabai announcing the death of Dadaji Bhikaji. The year was 1904, and she was not even forty. The deceased was the man she had refused to acknowledge as her husband. She had, of course, conceded that she was bound to remain single all her life. In that she had only acknowledged a legal bar, not accepted the man as her husband. Indeed, she had paid him off and earned her deliverance. Even that legal bar was gone now. She, as a widow, could now be free of the man.

We have no idea who thought of sending the telegram. Was it Dadaji's family? Or Rukhmabai's own? Whoever they were, and whatever their expectation in informing her urgently, no one would have expected her to do what she actually did. She got into a widow's garb – all white – and stayed in it till her last breath fifty-odd years later.

What would we make of that today? My own first reaction was one of disbelief and betrayal. I had in the course of my researches formed a veritable roster of distinguished Indians whose outstanding contributions in diverse fields had laid the foundations of new India. Rukhmabai outshone them all. Born in a hidebound society, denied schooling and used as a pawn in a petty plot to retain control over her property, she had surprised the world with her radical conception of women's freedom. And in asserting that freedom, she had shown the world a novel mode of resistance.

I just could not believe that my 'shero' had so tamely given in to tradition. The shero, suddenly, became an apostate. She, who as a twenty-year-old nobody had withstood the most formidable odds, had submitted when there was nothing – so I then thought – that could have held her back. It took me years to get over that feeling. Vestigially the feeling still lurks inside.

Then, slowly, I began to sense the moral tyranny of my own response. Whether she rose in defiance or conformed to tradition, Rukhmabai was always flesh and blood, subject to conflicting feelings, ideas, ideals, calculations. I had seen her only as the embodiment of an abstract cause.

If we see her as flesh and blood, and extend her the empathy due to a fellow human being, a very different understanding of her acceptance of widowhood ensues.

Rukhmabai, the doctor who quietly donned the widow's garb, was a far cry from Rukhmabai, the rebel determined to resist. The doctor's priorities and considerations in provincial Surat were very different from those of the rebel in metropolitan Bombay and London. So also was her understanding of what was practicable, desirable and necessary. What the others thought was of no consequence to the rebel. Her objective was to upset their settled ways of thinking and offer a radically different alternative. But the doctor in the provincial town could not ignore the others even as she tried to alter their ways of thinking.

For rebel Rukhmabai there was convergence between the demands of personal life and the larger cause. But Dr Rukhmabai was obliged to tailor her decisions and actions according to what people were likely to think of them. It is true that during the nine years that she had already been in their city, Surtis across the board had accorded her unqualified love and respect. Her history had not hampered their acceptance of her.

Then came the news of Dadaji's death. Rukhmabai had denied the legality of her marriage when her case came up before the Bombay High Court. The court had rejected her contention and she had felt compelled to accept a compromise. That done, the only sensible course for her was to move on. It was pointless to make an issue of her marital status. Happy to be addressed as 'Miss Rukhmabai', she would not object to being addressed as 'Mrs Rukhmabai'. Even in the UK, with its unreserved admiration for her, she was addressed as both 'Miss' and 'Mrs'.

Dadaji dead was hard to escape. Rukhmabai's marital status was back into the public gaze. Gone in an instant was the post-compromise freedom to lead the kind of single life she pleased. Hindus would not be Hindus if they ignored what she did as a widow. Even the relatively free Surtis would not take kindly to any deviance that affronted the dead husband. During the nine years she had been in the city, she had considerably weakened people's resistance to sending their women to her hospital. However, as against the Parsis and Muslims, the Hindus were still lukewarm in their response. One misstep now could risk that beginning.

Also, Rukhmabai had before her the sobering example of one she greatly loved and admired, Pandita Ramabai. Ramabai was only twenty-four when she donned the garb of a widow following her husband's death within two years of their marriage. Not long after that she embraced Christianity and was freed of all obligations as a Hindu. Still, she retained her Hindu widow's appearance and managed to be perceived as culturally a Hindu. This helped her reach out to Hindu women as one of their own. Ramabai even told the Education Commission that Hindu women who worked among their sisters must be correct in their morals and conduct.

Rukhmabai followed the call of duty when she defied tradition in the 1880s. She did the same when she conformed to tradition following Dadaji's death twenty years later.

This is one plausible explanation for Rukhmabai's acceptance of widowhood. Highlighting her self-efffacing commitment to public service, this explanation sees her as submitting to the system that she had rebelled against. Different from this, even contrary, there is another plausible explanation. Taking a dynamic view of her ideas and beliefs, this explanation sees her acceptance of widowhood as convergent with what she believed in at that time.

While writing the letters of 'A Hindu Lady', she was convinced of the truth of everything she said. But, then, came like a father figure Dewan Bahadur Raghunath Rao. He showed 'A Hindu Lady' that she had erred in dismissing the rishis and the shastras wholesale. And two days later, he came up with a powerful shastric defence of the besieged Rukhmabai. Turning the tables upon the orthodox, who assailed Rukhmabai for aping Western ways, Raghunath Rao accused them of not knowing their own tradition. In one brilliant move, he produced an authentic shastric justification for both Rukhmabai and Justice Pinhey. Confronting the orthodox with the legend of *vriddha kanya*, he wrote:

The legend is that there was a daughter of a Brahmin. She was well read. She was not disposed to be a devotee and desirous of final beatitude, but was looking for a husband. The bridegrooms who were willing to marry her and to whom her father was prepared to give her, proved her inferiors. Following Manu's view, viz., rather than marry an unequal partner, it is better to die a virgin, she continued a virgin till she grew very old. As she was going to commit suicide, Narada asked her what Lokas are secure for unmarried women. She then gave her hand to a Rishi, and having had sexual intercourse with him (as without it, there was no marriage) she died and went to heaven.[1]

Having shown that the spouse's consent (the principle on which rested Rukhmabai's case) and consummation – the basis of Pinhey's verdict – were essential for a valid Hindu marriage, Raghunath Rao hailed Rukhmabai as a martyr. Her persecution, he warned, confirmed the shastric prophecy 'that in this era persons not cognizant of the Law shall ascend royal seats and shall administer as law that which is no law'.[2]

For Rukhmabai, who had seen and suffered the hypocrisy of Hindu reformers, it was not easy to be persuaded by Raghunath Rao's defence of tradition. But, after the way he countered Hindu orthodoxy with his brilliant shastric defence of her resistance, she could not dismiss him as yet another of those reformers. Rather, Raghunath Rao forced her out of the one-dimensionality of her thinking.

Soon, Rukhmabai was surrounded by a galaxy of supporters who invoked the shastras to defend her defiance. One such, of course, was her own wise counsel, Telang. Another was Malabari. Feeling no less anguished and wrathful than did Raghunath Rao, Malabari wrote:

Just fancy the little rebel delivered into the hands of Dadaji Bhikhaji, his uncles, aunts, sisters and cousins. It makes one's blood curdle only to think of the outrage. If I had a child in that predicament, I would far rather she died before my eyes.

Malabari, too, swore by tradition as he defended Rukhmabai. When a 'usually sensible and impartial' writer lectured Rukhmabai on 'the wifely sacrifices' of Damayanti, Malabari gave the writer a lesson in the exegesis of tradition. Saying that he believed Damayanti's story to be true and not a mere figment of mythological imagination, he wrote:

> Damayanti accepted the husband of her choice, when she was old enough to exercise her judgment. Rukhmabai never lived with her husband since the sham marriage, did not know him, had no opportunity of studying his character ... Rukhmabai's nominal husband is said to have gone to the bad, ruining his mind and body for ever ...

Describing her as a 'nominal wife', Malabari asked: 'What right have we, as honest observers, to ask Rukhmabai to follow the example of Damayanti?'[3]

Rukhmabai realized that there were aspects of tradition and traditionalists of which she had known nothing. The realization helped her see things she had not seen before, or seen in an adverse light. She could see, for example, more than the traditional exterior of her widowed friend Shanta's father, R. G. Bhandarkar, who wanted his daughter to remarry. Similarly, more in widowed Ranade than the betrayal of the cause of social reform in marrying a virgin and not a widow. Still critical of Ranade's betrayal, she now valued his determination, in the teeth of domestic and social opposition, to educate his illiterate child-wife and make of her a fellow social reformer. There was also the example par excellence of Dr Atmaram Pandurang.

The Rukhmabai who received the news of Dadaji's death was not the raw rebellious writer of the letters of 'A Hindu Lady'. Her response to the news was in accord with her appreciation of the worth and beauty of tradition. We must understand, and not be surprised by, what she did.

Moreover, contrary to what is generally believed, the whole truth of Rukhmabai's relationship with Dadaji does not lie frozen in her decision to wash her hands of him. It was more complex and fluid. We have noted in chapter 1 that after his mother's death Dadaji left his father-in-law's house and began living with his villainous uncle, Narayan Dhurmaji. Soon thereafter occurred the harrowing event that led Rukhmabai to resolve to never again enter that house. She did not think of washing her hands of Dadaji then. She kept hoping that he might one day be a reformed person. She was even ready to try out a life with him – unreformed as he was – if he left his vile uncle and set up an independent establishment.

Washing her hands of him was not easy. She could not do it unilaterally. He, too, had to let it happen. Which he would not. Nor would, for a while, his uncle and the Hindu orthodoxy. He was an incubus she could not throw off. The longer he stuck to her, the deeper grew her anger, resentment and bitterness for him.

Then, at last, came the compromise and she left for London. Physical distance and passage of time helped her be at peace with herself. Having humbled the mighty combine of colonial law and Hindu orthodoxy, she, as a celebrity in London, could see that poor Dadaji had been a mere pawn. He was not worth her rancour. His proper place was in the realm of Rukhmabai's oblivion.

Then, soon after her return home, Dadaji, on an impulse, did something which, unwittingly, got him out of that oblivion. The Arya Mahila Samaj, of which Rukhmabai as a young girl had been secretary, organized a felicitation for her in a hall of Sheth Madhavdas Raghunathdas' large bungalow. The function was presided over by Dr Atmaram Pandurang. While great excitement prevailed among the invited guests and speaker after speaker extolled Rukhmabai's accomplishments, an unkempt man in his forties looked in furtively through a glass window. After the speeches were done, the man quietly beckoned to Nani, Rukhmabai's ten-year-old stepsister, and got her to let him hold in his hand her famous sister's medical 'degree', which had been put up for display at the function. That done, the man disappeared. This was Dadaji.

We are grateful to Mohini Varde for having recorded this incident.[4] There is no account of what happened thereafter. But Rukhmabai would certainly have come to know about the furtive visit. Even without moving her in a big way, it would have made her feel that, all said and done, he was not an evil man. He was, rather, an unfortunately circumstanced, vulnerable man whose life could as well have taken a happier turn.

Freed of his ghostly persona, Rukhmabai could now feel sorry for him and also be relieved that she was done with him.

Like her understanding of Hindu tradition and culture, her attitude towards Dadaji was not fixed and static. There is a telling detail in Mary L. Nind's first-hand description of Rukhmabai. Nind writes:

> She was simply clad in a blue cloth *sari* ... I noticed the striking absence of jewellery, with which the women and girls are usually so burdened. Her chief ornament was a gold chain, which she afterwards explained was put on her neck at her betrothal, and had never been removed.[5]

This description dates to March 1888, when Rukhmabai was disavowing her marriage. The disavowal is at odds with her wearing a chain that symbolized the disavowed marriage. Aggravating the oddity is her ready explication to a stranger of the significance of the symbol. It lends credence to the surmise that even as she repudiated them, she was vaguely ambivalent about the marriage and the man.

The fluctuations in Rukhmabai's attitude towards Hindu religion and culture, and towards Dadaji, call for a nuanced understanding of her acceptance of widowhood. It was in keeping with the logic of her life. For twenty years, from the moment of being forced into litigation to Dadaji's death, she had wished to be left alone. That is, indeed, how she had lived those years. Nonetheless, her defining identity – her title to fame and notoriety – was as a married woman. Now that the man responsible for that identity was gone, she had in reality become what she, in truth, had been: a widow.

What in that moment was going on in her mind? A great writer from her own time but a different culture, Dostoevsky, offers us an insight. He devotes the opening chapter of *The Brothers Karamazov* to describe the brief stormy marital life of Karamazov Sr. with a rich, rebellious and beautiful local lass, Adelaide Ivanova. Quick to sense there is nothing in the relationship, Adelaide runs away to Petersburg. As the husband plans to go to Petersburg to recover his wife, news reaches him of her death. Dostoevsky concludes the chapter thus:

… the story is that he ran out into the street and began shouting with joy … but others say he wept without restraint like a child … It is quite possible that both versions are true, that he rejoiced at his release and at the same time wept for her who released him. As a general rule, people, even the wicked, are much more naïve and simple-hearted than we suppose. And we ourselves are, too.

Coming from a distant time but Rukhmabai's own culture, another great writer anticipates Dostoevsky's insight. Describing pregnant Sita's exile in his *Raghuvansham*, Kalidasa shows Lakshman, ordered by Ram, taking Sita out on the pretext of fulfilling her desire to see sage Valmiki's ashram. Reaching there, Lakshman tells Sita the real purpose of their coming. She falls in a swoon. When she comes to, she asks Lakshman to tell 'that king' – not his brother, not her husband, not even Ram – that he was witness to the fire ordeal that had established her purity. Does it become his venerable dynasty that he should abandon her for some idle popular talk? Sita, it must be noted, does not simply tell the king. She also condemns him. For, the word she uses – *vachya* in Sanskrit – also carries the sense of condemnation. After she has condemned Ram, Sita's tone changes.

She comes up with reasons to justify his action, even saying that she is actually being punished for her own sins in the previous birth. She ends by telling Ram that, after she has given birth to his child, she would undertake a *tapasya* to have him as her consort again in the next birth.

Human response to life's momentous events is rarely, if ever, monochromatic. Least of all to death, which does strange things. Looking at how much Rukhmabai had to suffer on account of Dadaji, it may seem natural to conclude that rancour is all she could have felt for him. That, we have seen, was not so. In any case, if for no other reason than the final release his death brought her, she, for all her rancour, would also have shed a silent tear for him. To paraphrase Dostoevsky, she would have rejoiced in her liberation and also sorrowed for the man – Dadaji – whose death had liberated her.

Multiple though Rukhmabai's motivation in donning the widow's garb was, it presupposed a proud realization of being a Hindu. We have seen how this pride first entered rebellious Rukhmabai's awareness in the wake of her letters as 'A Hindu Lady'. That pride had in the intervening twenty years deepened enough for the erstwhile rebel to submit to tradition of her own volition. From now on, the inner conviction and the outer appearance would enforce each other. The quiet, indefatigable rebel of old would be a quiet, proud Hindu henceforth.

Keeping up the tradition of those, like Raghunath Rao, who had taught her what it was to be a proud Hindu, she would not turn a blind eye to the evils plaguing her society. But she would not let her Hindu pride make her demand religious-cultural autarchy. As before, she would retain her faith in legislation and expect the British to be true to their civilizing mission. Thus, in a paper on the anti-women practice of 'purdah', she wrote in 1929:

A sweeping change through legislation would finally be a simpler matter than cautious attempts at compromise. Turkey has completely abolished purdah by legislation. A very slow and laborious method has often been suggested and occasionally followed, of attacking this institution by education, by a method of house-to-house visiting in order to teach Moslem girls, and by holding classes under secluded conditions and at times when it is possible for these girls to leave their domestic work. But the method is slow, laborious and very costly in proportion to the results obtained.[6]

The paper on 'purdah' may suggest a continuity in Rukhmabai's concern about the evils that held back women's progress, and in her strategy for doing away with those evils. But it is an aberration. For, while in service, she was confined, as a matter of principle, to her work as a doctor and, in retirement, to the privacy of her home.

She lived a quiet retired life and passed on quietly.

Notes

Introduction

1. 'The Problem of Social Reform in Modern India: The Study of a Case', in S. C. Malik, ed., *Dissent, Protest, and Reform in Indian Civilization* (Simla: Indian Institute of Advanced Study, 1977), 250–67.

2. Richard P. Tucker, *Ranade and the Roots of Indian Nationalism* (Bombay: Popular Prakashan, 1977, first published 1972), 213–14.

3. Sudhir Chandra, 'Whose Laws? Notes on a Legitimising Myth of the Colonial Indian State', *Studies in History*, New Series, vol. 8, no. 2, August 1992, 187–211.

4. Meera Kosambi, 'The Meeting of the Twain: The Cultural Confrontation of Three Women in Nineteenth Century Maharashtra', *Indian Journal of Gender Studies*, Centre for Women's Development Studies, vol. 1, no. 1, 1–22.

5. Antoinette Burton, *At the Heart of the Empire: Indians and the Colonial Encounter in Late-Victorian Britain* (Berkeley: University of California Press, 1998), 18.

6. Tanika Sarkar, 'Rhetoric against Age of Consent: Resisting Colonial Reason and Death of a Child-Wife', *Economic & Political Weekly*, vol. 28, no. 36, 4 September 1993, 1873.

7. Swati Save, *My Dreams are not for Sale* (Bloomington, Indiana: Xlibris Corporation, 2012), 62–3.

8. 'Letter to editor', *The Times*, 9 April 1887.

9. Wikipedia cites Helen Rappaport, *Queen Victoria: A Biographical Companion* (ABC-CLIO, 2003), 429, for the supposed dissolution of Rukhmabai's marriage.

10. Sarkar, 'Rhetoric against Age of Consent', 1870.

11. *Home Department, Judicial Proceedings,* June 1887, no. 189–92 (National Archives of India).

12. Ibid.

13. Tanika Sarkar, 'The Hindu Wife and the Hindu Nation: Domesticity and Nationalism in Nineteenth Century Bengal', *Studies in History,* vol. 8, no. 2, New Series, 1992, 229, 232.

14. Burton, *At the Heart of the Empire,* note 140, 205–6.

15. Sudhir Chandra, *Enslaved Daughters: Colonialism, Law and Women's Rights* (Oxford University Press, February 2008), 10.

16. Deirdre David, *Intellectual Women and Victorian Patriarchy: Harriet Martineau, Barrett Browning, George Eliot* (London: Palgrave Macmillan, 1987), 237.

17. Richard Sorabji, *Opening Doors: The Untold Story of Cornelia Sorabji, Reformer, Lawyer and Champion of Women's Rights in India* (London: I.B. Tauris, 2010).

1. Beginnings in Sadness

1. Mary L. Nind, 'Rukhmabai in Her Home', *Christian Advocate,* vol. 64, no. 11, 14 March 1889, 164.

2. *Times of India,* 14 August 1884.

3. 'Rukhmabai's "Reply" to Dadaji's 'Exposition', *Times of India,* 29 June 1887.

4. Rukhmabai, 'Infant Marriage and Enforced Widowhood', *Times of India,* 26 June 1885.

5. *Times of India,* 13 March 1886.

6. *Kesari,* 19 April 1887.

7. Tarabai Shinde, *Stree-Purush Tulana* (Sudhir Prakashan, 2018).

8. Sudhir Chandra, *Enslaved Daughters: Colonialism, Law and Women's Rights* (Oxford University Press, February 2008), 242.

9. Mridula Ramanna, *Western Medicine and Public Health in Colonial Bombay 1845–1895* (Orient Longman: New Delhi, 2002), 45.

10. Kavitha Rao, *Lady Doctors: The Untold Stories of India's First Women in Medicine* (Chennai: Westland, July 2021); Kavitha Rao, Book excerpt,

'This book recovers the stories of India's first women doctors, often ignored by history', *Scroll*, 2 July 2021. Available: https://scroll.in/article/999008/this-book-recovers-the-stories-of-indias-first-women-doctors-often-ignored-by-history.

11. 'Rukhmabai to Miss Carlisle, 17 February 1887', *The Times*, 9 April, 1887.

12. *Bombay Gazette*, 30 July 1887.

13. Rukhmabai, 'Letter of "A Hindu Lady"', *Times of India*, 26 June 1885.

14. Sarojini Sharangpani, *Mala He Lagna Manya Nahi* (Pune: Shri Vidya Prakashan, 1983) 33–4.

15. Nora Scott, *An Indian Journal* (London: Radcliffe Press, 1994), 43.

16. Rukhmabai, 'Letter of "A Hindu Lady"', *Times of India*, 26 June 1885.

17. Scott, *An Indian Journal*, 87.

18. Ibid., 42.

19. Ibid.

20. Rukhmabai's letter of 17 Feb. 1887 to Miss Carlisle, published in *The Times*, 9 April 1887.

21. Rukhmabai, 'Letter of "A Hindu Lady"', *Times of India*, 26 June 1885.

22. Rukhmabai, 'Letter to editor', *The Times*, 9 April 1887.

23. 'Dadaji's Exposition', *Times of India*, 19 April 1887.

24. 'Rukhmabai's "Reply" to Dadaji's "Exposition"', *Times of India*, 29 June 1887.

25. Ibid.

26. *Times of India*, 14 August 1884.

27. Rukhmabai, 'Letter to editor', *The Times*, 9 April 1887.

28. Meera Kosambi, *A Fragmented Feminism: The Life and Letters of Anandibai Joshee* (London: Routledge, 2020), 154.

29. Ibid., 153–4.

30. Caroline Healey Dall, *The Life of Dr Anandibai Joshee, A kinswoman of the Pundita Ramabai*, (Boston: Robert Brothers, 1888), 138.

31. Margaret Todd, M. D., *The Life of Sophia Jex-Blake* (London: Macmillan and Co., 1918), 494.

32. Scott, *An Indian Journal*, 118.

33. Ibid., 118–19.

34. Ibid., 118.

35. Rukhmabai, 'Letter to editor', *The Times*, 9 April 1887.

36. 'Rukhmabai's "Reply" to Dadaji's "Exposition"', *Times of India*, 29 June 1887.

37. *Clifton & Redland Free Press*, 11 July 1890.

2. Quiet Making of a Rebel

1. Mohini Varde, *Dr Rakhmabai: An Odyssey* (New Delhi: Minerva Press, 2000), 25.

2. 'Rukhmabai's "Reply" to Dadaji's "Exposition"', *Times of India*, 29 June 1887.

3. 'My Education', in Meera Kosambi (tr. and ed.), *Feminist Vision or 'Treason Against Men'?: Kashinai Kanitkar and the Engendering of Marathi Literature*, (Ranikhet: Permanent Black, 2008), 54.

4. Varde, *Dr Rakhmabai: An Odyssey*, 97.

5. Edythe Lutzker, *Edith Pechey Phipson, M.D.: The Story of England's Foremost Pioneering Woman Doctor* (New York: Exposition Press, 1973), 207–08.

6. L. Martindale, *A Woman Surgeon* (London: Victor Gollancz, 1951), 30.

7. Lutzker, op. cit., 207–08.

8. *Times of India*, 19 September 1885.

9. *Times of India*, 3 October 1885.

10. *Indu Prakash*, 21 September 1885.

11. 'Letter to editor', *The Times*, 9 April 1887.

12. *The New Review*, September 1890, 263–69.

13. *Indian Spectator*, 1 November 1885.

3. To the High Court

1. Scott, *An Indian Journal*, 40.

2. *Times of India*, 19 September 1885.

3. 'Letter to editor', *The Times*, 9 April 1887.

4. Dadaji, 'An Exposition of Some of the Facts of the Case Dadaji Vs Rakhmabai', *Times of India*, 19 April 1887.

5. 'Letter to editor', *The Times*, 9 April 1887.
6. Dadaji, 'An Exposition of Some of the Facts of the Case Dadaji Vs Rakhmabai', *Times of India*, 19 April 1887.
7. 'Letter to editor', *The Times*, 9 April 1887.
8. Dadaji, 'An Exposition of Some of the Facts of the Case Dadaji Vs Rakhmabai', *Times of India*, 19 April 1887.
9. Scott, *An Indian Journal*, 40.
10. Priyanka Lad and V. N. Nail, 'Kashinath Trimbak Telang 1850-1893: A Memoir', Bombay, 1951, 49.

4. Rukhmabai Triumphs

1. *Indian Spectator*, 23 December, 1894.

5. The Magic of Moral Defiance

1. *Times of India*, 30 September 1885.
2. *Bombay Guardian*, excerpted in the *Civil and Military Gazette*, 12 October 1885.
3. *Native Opinion*, 27 September 1885.
4. *Kesari*, 19 April 1887.
5. *Hindoo Patriot*, 4 and 18 April 1887.
6. *Indian Spectator*, 27 March 1887.
7. *Prachar*, vol. 3, 1293–94, B.S., 390–99.
8. *Home Department, Judicial Proceedings*, June 1887, nos. 189-92 (National Archives of India).
9. *Home Department, Judicial Proceedings*, September 1887, no. 299 (National Archives of India).
10. *Indian Spectator*, 10 July 1887.
11. *Bombay Gazette*, 26 September 1887.
12. *Indian Daily News*, 3 August 1887.
13. *Times of India*, 24 March 1887.
14. Varde, *Dr Rakhmabai: An Odyssey*, 102.
15. C. Amy Dawson, *Idylls of Womanhood* (London: William Heinmann, 1892), 58–9.

6. Another Brave Decision

1. Lutzker, op. cit., 208.

7. Six Years in England

1. 'An Interview with Mrs Eva McLaren', *The Woman's Signal*, 31 May 1894.
2. *Englishwoman's Review*, 15 January 1890.
3. *Times of India*, 19 August 1924.
4. Hannah Whitall Smith, 'A Hindu Heroine. A Sketch of Rukhmabai', *The Woman's Signal*, 25 October 1894.
5. Ibid.
6. *The Times, St. James's Gazette*, 29 April 1889; Supplement to the *Cheltenham Chronicle*, 4 May 1889.
7. *The Madras Weekly Mail*, 17 January 1895.
8. *The Australasian*, 12 October 1889.
9. *Indian Female Evangelist*, 1 October 1889.
10. *The Australasian*, 12 October 1889.
11. Burton, *At the Heart of the Empire*, 125.
12. 'Letter to editor', *Times of India*, 9 April 1887.
13. *Indian Female Evangelist*, 1 January 1890.
14. *Clifton & Redland Free Press*, 11 July 1890.
15. *The Queen*, 19 July 1890.
16. Letter of 8 October 1889, quoted in *At the Heart of the Empire*, 127.
17. Letter of 2 February 1890, Ibid., 142.
18. *Clifton & Redland Free Press*, 11 July 1890.
19. Isabel Thorne, *Sketch of the Foundation and Development of the London School of Medicine for Women* (1905), 30.
20. *Indian Female Evangelist*, 1 January 1890.
21. Letter of 2 October 1889, in Suparna Gooptu, *Cornelia Sorabji: India's Pioneer Woman Lawyer* (New Delhi: Oxford University Press, 2006), 6.
22. Mary L. Nind, 'Rukhmabai in Her Home,' *Christian Advocate*, 14 March 1889.

23. *The Northern Whig*, 7 October 1891.

24. Burton, *At the Heart of the Empire*, 123.

25. Dr Louisa Garrett Anderson, *Elizabeth Garrett Anderson, 1836-1917* (London: Faber and Faber Ltd., 1939), 50 in Karen Michaelsen, 'Becoming "Medical Women"', 13.

26. Sophia Jex-Blake, *Medical Women* (Legare Street Press, 2023), 79.

27. *The Northern Whig*, 7 October 1891.

28. *The British Medical Journal*, vol. 2, no. 1765, 6 October 1894, 788.

29. *Minutes of Evidence Taken before the Select Committee on Metropolitan Hospitals, &c.* (London: Eyre & Spottiswoode, 1890), 298–300.

30. Dr Margaret Todd, *Life of Dr Sophia Jex-Blake* (London: Macmillan, 1918), 504.

31. Varde, *Dr Rakhmabai: An Odyssey*, 113.

32. Burton, *At the Heart of the Empire*, 142–43.

33. Ibid., note 158, 225.

34. Scott, *An Indian Journal*, 80.

35. Burton, *At the Heart of the Empire*, 142.

36. Richard Sorabji, *Opening Doors: The Untold Story of Cornelia Sorabji, Reformer, Lawyer and Champion of Women's Rights in India* (Penguin India, 2010), 31–32.

37. Burton, *At the Heart of the Empire*, 124–27.

38. Sorabji, *Opening Doors*, 32.

39. Hannah Whitall Smith, 'A Hindu Heroine: A Sketch of Rukhmabai', *The Woman's Signal*, 25 October 1894.

8. Quiet Service

1. 'The Sphere of Indian Women in Medical Work in India', in Evelyn C. Gedge and Mithan Choksi (eds.), *Women in Modern India: Fifteen Papers by Indian Women Writers* (Bombay: D.B. Taraporewala Sons & Co., 1929), 51.

2. Ibid., 61.

3. George Kittredge, *A Short History of the "Medical Women for India" Fund of Bombay* (Bombay: Education Society Press, 1889), 1–2.

4. W. W. Hunter, 'A Female Medical Profession for India', *The Contemporary Review*, August 1889, 207.

5. World Medical Journal, vol. 2, no. 1, 1964, 35.

6. Louisa Martindale, *A Woman Surgeon* (London: Gollancz, 1951), 60–1.

7. *Times of India*, 23 October 1915.

8. 'Rukhmabai, L. R. C. P. &S., M. D. (Brux.), Medical Officer in Charge, Women's Hospital, Surat, with the kind assistance of B. H. Bennett, Major, L. M. S., Civil Surgeon 'A Case of Myxoma Operated upon at the Women's Hospital, Surat', *The Indian Medical Gazette*, May 1909, 180.

9. *Times of India*, 23 October 1915.

10. Varde, *Dr Rakhmabai: An Odyssey*, 141.

11. *Times of India*, 23 October 1915.

12. Varde, *Dr Rakhmabai: An Odyssey*, 144–6.

9. Widow's Garb

1. *A Letter Addressed to the Honourable W.W. Hunter, Ll. D., CIE, on the Subject of Hindu Re-marriage by Dewan Bahadur R. Raghunath Rao* (Madras, 1885), 5.

2. *Indian Spectator*, 13 March 1887.

3. *Indian Spectator*, 1 November 1885.

4. Varde, *Dr Rakhmabai: An Odyssey*, 120–21.

5. 'Rukhmabai in Her Home', *Christian Advocate*, 14 March 1889.

6. Evelyn C. Gedge and Mithan Choksi, eds. *Women in Modern India: Fifteen Papers by Modern Indian Writers* (Bombay: Taraporewala Sons & Co. 1929), 147–48.

Index